HEALING THROUGH NATURAL FOODS

H. K. Bakhru

By the same author:

A Complete Handbook of Nature Cure (Revised & Enlarged Edition)

Diet Cure For Common Ailments

A Handbook Of Natural Beauty

Nature Cure For Children's Diseases

Naturopathy For The Elderly

Indian Spices And Condiments As Natural Healers

Foods That Heal

Herbs That Heal

Natural Home Remedies For Common Ailments

Vitamins That Heal

Conquering Cancer Naturally

HEALING THROUGH NATURAL FOODS

H. K. Bakhru

JAICO PUBLISHING HOUSE
Mumbai • Delhi • Bangalore
Kolkata • Hyderabad • Chennai

HEALING THROUGH NATURAL FOODS
ISBN 81-7224-860-1

First Jaico Impression: 2000
Second Jaico Impression: 2001

Published by:
Jaico Publishing House
121, M.G. Road
Mumbai - 400 001.

Printed by:
Paras Printing Press
123, Adhyaru Ind. Estate,
Sunmill Compound,
Lower Parel, Mumbai - 400 013.

ABOUT THE AUTHOR

Dr. H.K. Bakhru enjoys a countrywide reputation as an expert naturopath and a prolific writer. His well-researched articles on nature cure, health, nutrition and herbs appear regularly in various newspapers and magazines and they bear the stamp of authority.

A diploma holder in Naturopathy, all his current twelve books on nature cure, nutrition and herbs titled, *A Complete Handbook of Nature Cure (Revised and enlarged edition), Diet Cure For Common Ailments, A Handbook of Natural Beauty, Nature Cure For Children's Diseases, Naturopathy For The Elderly, Healing Through Natural Foods, Indian Spices And Condiments As Natural Healers, Foods That Heal, Herbs That Heal, Natural Home Remedies for Common Ailments, Vitamins that Heal* and *Conquering Cancer Naturally* have been highly appreciated by the public and repeatedly reprinted. His first-named book has been awarded first prize in the category 'Primer on Naturopathy for Healthy Living' by the jury of judges at the Book Prize Award scheme, organized by National Institute of Naturopathy, an autonomous body under Govt. of India, Ministry of health.

Dr. Bakhru began his career with the Indian Railways, with a first class first postgraduate degree in History from Lucknow University in 1949. He retired in October 1984 as the Chief Public Relations Officer of the Central Railway in Bombay, having to his credit 35 years of distinguished service in Public Relations with the Indian Railways and the Railway Board.

An associate member of all India Alternative Medical Practitioner's Association and a member of the Nature Cure Practitioners' Guild in Mumbai, Dr. Bakhru has made extensive studies on natural methods of treating diseases and herbalism. He has been honoured with 'Lifetime Achievement Award', 'Gem of Alternative Medicines' award and a gold medal in Diet Therapy by the Indian Board of Alternative Medicines - Calcutta, in recognition of his dedication and outstanding contributions in the field of Alternative Medicines. The Board, which is affiliated with the Open International University for Complementary Medicines, established under World Health Organisation and recognised by the United Nations Peace University, has also appointed him as its Honorary Advisor. Dr. Bakhru has also been honoured by Nature Cure Practitioners' Guild, Mumbai with Nature Cure Appreciation Award for his services to Naturopathy.

Dr. Bakhru has founded a registered Public Charitable Trust, known as D.H. Bakhru Foundation for help to the poor and needy. He has been donating Rs. 25,000 every year to this trust from his income as writer and author.

Dr. Bakhru spends his retired life, devoting all his time to the furtherance of the cause of nature cure and charitable activities under the auspices of the Trust. He is willing to offer advice to those who come to seek his help for solving their health problems. He can be contacted at:

Dr. H. K. Bakhru
Bldg-9, Flat No. 602,
Mhada HIG Complex,
Oshiwara, Andheri(W).
Mumbai-400 053.
Telephone: 6398779, Fax: 6398825
E-mail: hkbakhru@hotmail.com

❀ ❀ ❀

CONTENTS

Preface

There is a growing awareness today about the efficacy of alternative medicines for the maintenance of good health and for the prevention and treatment of diseases. More and more people are now turning to them for solving their health problems. Surveys show that at least one-third of people in America use alternative medicines in some form or the other at present. Diet therapy is undoubtedly the best and the safest form of alternative medicines.

Latest researches indicate that foods affect cellular behavior, which may lead to health or disease. They also show which foods, are likely to alleviate specific diseases. These researches have enabled a large number of people to become aware of the preventive and healing powers of specific foods. Many of them all over the world have been treating them-selves successfully of their long-standing illnesses by giving up harmful foods that caused them as well as poisonous drugs used for their treatment. They have now resorted to nutritious and well-balanced diet, with emphasis on specific foods found to contain valuable natural drugs. Some of them have already achieved great success and have freed themselves of many dread diseases. They are now enjoying health and happy lives and are living proofs that correct eating can save mankind from all kinds of diseases.

The various medicinal properties attributed to different foods as mentioned in this book have been scientifically tested and established by research studies. These studies have confirmed beyond doubt the healing and preventive powers of natural foods.

NATURAL FOODS AS MIRACLE MEDICINE

Hippocrates (460-357 BC), the father of medicine said, "Let food be the medicine and let medicine be the food." The former part of the sentence is for the sick, the latter is for the healthy. For the sick, positive natural foods are the true natural drugs and not commercially marketed drugs, which are not conducive to health as all of them have adverse side effects. For the healthy, natural foods are the means of freedom from disease. Hippocrates fully believed that natural foods have unlimited power to sustain health and restore it when lost.

There is hardly a health problem or natural bodily process that is not influenced in some way or the other by the foods we eat. There has been an increase in the variety and frequency of diseases in proportion to the process of the degeneration of foodstuffs through refining. Researches carried out on separate varieties of fruits, vegetables and other foodstuffs, have shown that natural foods possess the property of curing almost every kind of disease. These researches indicate that certain specific foods can serve as powerful natural drugs like laxatives, antibiotics, antidepressants, antiulcerants, analgesics, tranquillizers, cholesterol reducers, cancer fighters, fertility agents, antihyper-tensives, diuretics, anti-inflammatory agents, blood vessels dilators and so on.

Food can thus be redefined as miracle medicine that we can use in preventing and treating diseases of all kinds and in boosting mental and physical energy, vigour and well being. The adoption of sensible eating of natural foods can thus free mankind from all diseases. Natural foods, contain all essential vitamins, minerals, trace elements and other constituents, whereas in refined foods they are largely absent.

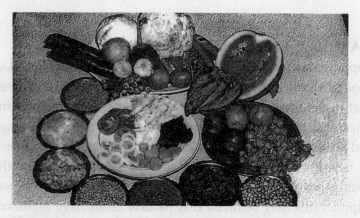

Natural foods like seeds, nuts and grains, vegetables and fruits can serve as powerful natural drugs.

This book describes in great detail the specific pharmacological action of specific natural foods, as established by scientific studies. This information can serve as a guide to the readers to treat common diseases through use of specific foods, besides adopting a well balanced natural diet consisting of 80 per cent of alkaline forming foods like fruits and vegetables and 20 per cent of acid forming foods like cereals and pulses. It would however be advisable to consult a biologically-oriented doctor or an expert naturopath in case of serious illnesses.

CHAPTER 1

ANTI-BACTERIAL FOODS

In 1858, Louis Pasteur first discovered the germ theory of the disease. He demonstrated that microbes were the cause of the decomposition of foods. He showed that the anthrax bacterium caused the dreaded disease of the same name, and discovered that small viruses cause rabies.

In the first paper in which Louis Pasteur published his discoveries of the germ theory of disease, he also mentioned that garlic had antibiotic property. He noted that bacteria died when exposed to garlic. Thus, garlic was the first antibiotic food that was used against germs, within years of this discovery. Subsequently studies were conducted to ascertain anti-bacterial activity of various other foods that can be used as antibiotic against germs.

FOODS THAT FIGHT INFECTIONS

Cabbage, Carrot, Clove, Coconut, Cumin Seeds, Curd, Drumstick, Eggplant Leaves, Garlic, Ginger, Honey, Lemon, Lime, Mango, Margosa, Onion, Pineapple, Radish, Sage and Turmeric.

Cabbage

The cabbage is one of the most high-rated leafy vegetables and is a marvelous food. It is grown for its enlarged edible, terminal buds and is eaten all over the world. It is excellent as a muscle builder and cleanser. This vegetable is

3

chiefly valued for its high mineral and vitamin contents and alkaline salts.

Cabbage is an antibiotic food and it possesses anti-bacterial powers. It can destroy a variety of bacteria in test tubes, including H. Pylori bacteria, which is now considered as a cause of stomach ulcers. Liberal intake of the fresh juice of this vegetable has thus been found very valuable in both gastric and duodenal ulcers. About 180 ml of this juice should be taken, mixed with a teaspoon of honey, twice daily in treating these conditions. This juice can also be used beneficially in treating some other infectious diseases like obstructive jaundice and bladder infection.

Carrot

The carrot, a popular vegetable, is a highly protective food. It is rich in beta-carotene and other food ingredients. It is an antioxidant and a powerful cleansing food. This vegetable is rich in alkaline elements, which purify and revitalise the blood. It nourishes the entire system and helps in the maintenance of acid-alkaline balance in the body.

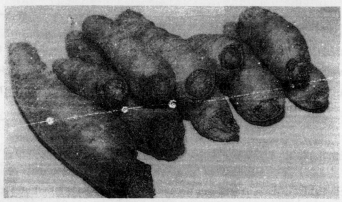

Carrot is one of the most important infection-fighting foods, with wide protective powers.

Carrot is one of the most important infection-fighting foods, with wide protective powers. It is especially valuable in the form of juice, which is a natural solvent for ulcerous and cancerous conditions. It is resistant to infections and does most efficient work in conjunction with the adrenal glands. This juice helps prevent infections of eyes, throat, tonsils and sinuses as well as of the respiratory organs generally.

Carrots are also valuable in the elimination of threadworms from children, as it is offensive to all parasites. A small cup of grated carrot taken every morning, with no other food added to the meal, can clear these worms quickly.

Carrot is best for health when eaten raw. It can be taken either whole, sliced or grated in salad. The skin should not be scraped off but should be thoroughly cleaned, as its mineral contents are very close to the skin. The leaves of this vegetable, which are usually discarded, are highly nourishing and health-building food.

Clove

Clove, one of the most popular spices, is the dried unopened flower bud obtained from a handsome, middle-sized, evergreen tree. It is of great medicinal value as an antiseptic food. This property arises from the volatile oil contained in it. Its use in case of toothache reduces pain and also helps decrease infection. Clove oil, applied to the cavity in a decayed tooth, relieves toothache.

Cloves are also effective in treating cholera infection. About four grams of this spice should be boiled in three litres of water until half the water has evaporated. This water, taken in draughts, will check severe symptoms of the disease.

Coconut

The coconut is known as a wonder food. It is a near perfect diet, as it contains almost all the essential nutrients needed by the human body. The water of the tender green coconut, generally known as mineral water, is an antibacterial food. This water is especially valuable in cholera infection. About 250 to 375 ml. of this water, mixed with a teaspoon of fresh limejuice, should be given orally to the patient. It rectifies the electrolyte balance and neutralises the acidosis of the blood. Green coconut water is a known source of potassium rich fluids and since cholera patients can almost invariably take oral fluids following initial correction of shock and acidosis, intake of coconut water has been found highly beneficial for them. Coconut is also an ancient remedy for expelling all kinds of intestinal worms. A tablespoon of the freshly ground coconut should be taken at breakfast, followed by 30 to 60 ml of castor oil mixed with 250 to 375 ml of lukewarm milk after three hours. The process may be repeated till the cure is complete.

Cumin Seeds

Cumin seeds are one of the oldest spices, known since Biblical times. They are a powerful antibacterial food. They are rich source of thymol, which is an anthelmintic against hookworm infections and also as an antiseptic in many proprietary preparations. Dilute cumin water is an antiseptic beverage and very useful in common cold and fevers. To prepare cumin water, a teaspoon of cumin seed is added to boiling water, which is allowed to simmer for a few seconds and set aside to cool. If the cold is associated with sore throat, a few small pieces of dry ginger should be added to the water. This soothes throat irritation.

Curd

An Ancient Wonder food, curd or yoghurt is strongly antibacterial. Although it has a nutritive content similar to fresh milk, it has extensive special values for therapeutic purposes. During the process of making curd, bacteria convert milk into curd, and predigest milk protein. These bacteria then inhibit the growth of hostile or illness-causing bacteria inside the intestinal tract and promote beneficial bacteria needed for digestion. Buttermilk, which has same nutritive and curative values as curd, is prepared by churning curd and adding some water, removing the fat in the form of butter.

The germs, which give rise to infection and inflammation such as those, that cause appendicitis, diarrhoea and dysentery, cannot thrive in the presence of lactic acid found in curd and buttermilk. A daily intake of 225 grams of curd reduces colds and other upper respiratory infections in humans.

Drumstick

The drumstick is a fairly common vegetable grown all over India. It is valued mainly for the tender pod. It is antibacterial and a wonderful cleanser. The leaves of drumstick tree are especially beneficial in the treatment of many ailments due to their various medicinal properties. They are full of iron and used as food.

Drumstick soup prepared from leaves and flowers, as well as boiled drumsticks, is a very valuable antibiotic food. It has been found highly beneficial in preventing infections of all kinds such as that of the throat, chest and skin. This is because drumstick has antibacterial properties very much like penicillin and other antibiotics.

Eggplant Leaves

The eggplant, also known as brinjal, is botanically a fruit but extensively used as a culinary vegetable. It is wholesome and is grown all over India in all seasons of the year. This vegetable is an antibacterial and antiphlegmatic food.

The leaves of this plant are an antibacterial food. They are an effective medicine for several infectious and viral diseases. They can be beneficially used in the treatment of whooping cough, bronchitis, congestion in the lungs and difficult expectoration. Half a tablespoonful of fresh juice mixed with honey should be given three times daily in treating these conditions. The juice extracted from the root may also be mixed with leaf juice to increase its medicinal effects.

Garlic

The garlic, a garden vegetable of the onion family, has been cultivated from time immemorial. It has been variously described as a food, a herb, a medicinal plant, an antiseptic, and a magical antidote to evil by various people at different times throughout the ages. It is an important condiment crop.

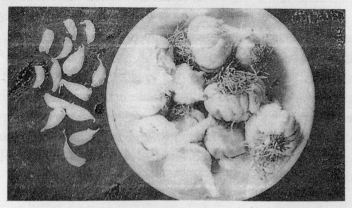

Garlic was the first antibiotic food that was used against germs.

Garlic is one of the nature's strongest, antibacterial foods. Tests show that garlic kills or cripples at least 72 infection bacteria that spread diarrhoea, dysentery, tuberculosis and encephalitis, among other diseases.

Dr. Tariq Abdullah, a prominent Indian garlic researcher from the Akbar Clinic and Research Center in Panama city, Florida, said in the August 1987 issue of Prevention magazine: "Garlic has the broadest spectrum of any antimicrobial substance that we know of its antibacterial, anti-fungal, antiparasitic, anti-protozoan, antiviral." Researchers have even found raw garlic extract in rats were more effective than the common antibiotic tetracycline.

Infections like cholera, typhoid and dysentery caused by organisms can readily become resistant to antibiotic therapy. They are all life threatening and are still endemic in many countries today. Garlic is one of the most effective remedies for these disorders. Its action has been confirmed against the specific classes of bacteria responsible for these diseases in laboratory test.

Garlic has another important benefit. Antibiotics usually kill all bacteria in the human system, including some that are beneficial. This can create many new problems. After a short while, harmful bacteria may occupy the vacant sites left by the beneficial bacteria, which have been removed. It is quite common for patient on antibiotic therapy to find that another infection, such as candida, takes over. A sore mouth or throat can often be the sign that a secondary infection of another type has occurred after a course of antibiotic. In case of garlic, while the harmful bacteria may be successfully eradicated, the beneficial bacteria do not seem to get eliminated.

Garlic works as an antibiotic in various forms. Raw garlic taken orally kills infectious bacteria in the intestines directly. Crushed garlic in water as a douche or a clove of garlic inserted in vagina kills infectious organisms in the vaginal tract. Garlic nose drops directly kill the viruses, which cause cold or influenza. Bacteria and viruses in the lungs and bronchial tract can be killed by Garlic's sulphur compounds, absorbed either through food, or inhalation or poultices, and then excreted through the lungs.

According to Dr. F.W.Crosman, an eminent physician, garlic is a marvelous remedy for pneumonia, if given in sufficient quantities. This physician used garlic for many years in pneumonia, and said that in no instance did it fail to bring down the temperature as well as the pulse and respiration, within 48 hours. Garlic juice can also be applied externally to the chest with beneficial results, as it is an irritant and rubefacient.

Garlic can also be used beneficially in the treatment of earache and discharge from the ear arising from middle-ear infection. A few cloves should be warmed and mashed with salt. This mixture should be wrapped in a piece of woolen cloth and placed on the painful ear. Simultaneously, two or three cloves of garlic should be chewed daily for few days.

Garlic oil is also a popular remedy for earache. If garlic oil is not available, a few peeled cloves of garlic can be put in a tablespoon of any sweet oil, except groundnut oil. This oil should be heated, till the oil becomes brown with charred garlic pieces. The oil should then be filtered and cooled and a few drops should be put in the affected ear for immediate relief.

Ginger

Ginger is a root vegetable and a spice. It is being used in India from Vedic period and is called *Maha-Aushadi*, meaning the great medicine. It contributes greatly towards health and is regarded as a food medicine for several ailments.

Ginger is an antibiotic and helps fight infection. It has been used for centuries to treat many infectious diseases like cholera, diarrhoea and chest congestion. Its use has been found especially effective in whooping cough. A teaspoon of the fresh ginger juice, mixed with a cup of fenugreek decoction and honey to taste, acts as an expectorant and diaphoretic in this disease. The fenugreek decoction can be made by boiling one teaspoon of seeds in 250 ml of water till it is reduced to half.

Honey

Honey contains strong antibiotic property. It is very beneficial in case of many infections. For throat infection, gargling with honey water relieves inflammation. This gargle is also an excellent remedy for hoarseness brought about by local infection of the throat.

Another recipe for throat infection and hoarseness is to grind well black pepper, asafoetida, Indian mustard and saffror in equal quantities and make pills by adding a little honey to it. One pill may be put in the mouth and sucked. After sometime the voice become as clear as before.

Honey is the best medicine for oral ulceration and sore tongue, which are very painful. These conditions may result from fungal or bacterial infection due to poor oral hygiene. The patient finds difficulty in eating, drinking and talking, especially when the ulcers are present at the angle of lips. For immediate relief from this condition, 20 grams of borax should be ground to fine powder and mixed thoroughly with 150 grams of honey and 10 grams of glycerin. This mixture should be applied locally over the ulcers two or three times daily. Proper oral hygiene is necessary with this treatment.

The use of honey has also been found very beneficial in the treatment of middle ear infection, known as Otitis Media in

Medical Parlance. This disease is characterised by infection of the ear leading to pus discharge through perforated eardrum. This condition can be treated by instilling honey in the ear. This will drain out all the pus and will lead to early healing of the middle ear infection. Later on, even the perforated eardrum will heal up automatically.

Lemon

The lemon is an important fruit of citrus group. It ranks high as a health food. The various parts of lemon used for medicinal purposes are rind of the ripe fruit, essential oil of the rind and expressed juice of the ripe fruit.

Lemon is antibacterial food and is highly beneficial in the treatment of infectious diseases. For throat infection, a ripe unpeeled lemon should be roasted slowly until it begins to crack open. One teaspoon of the juice with a little honey should be taken once every hour. In the alternative, the same juice of the roasted lemon should be mixed in a glass of boiled water and taken flavoured with honey. It should be sipped slowly.

Lemon contains wonderful anticholera property. Lemon juice can kill cholera bacilli within a very short time. It is a very effective and reliable preventive against cholera during the epidemic. For this purpose, it can be taken in the form of sweetened or salted beverages. Taking of lemon with food as a daily routine also prevents cholera.

Lime

Lime, like lemon, is an important citrus fruit and is very popular throughout the tropics. The juice of this fruit, which is used as medicine since ancient times, possesses antibacterial property. Its use has been found beneficial in infections like cold, tonsillitis and cystitis or bladder infection. For cold and tonsillitis, a fresh lime should be squeezed in a glass of warm water, to which a teaspoon of honey and a quarter teaspoon of common salt may be added. It should then be sipped slowly.

In case of bladder infection, a teaspoon of limejuice should be put in 180 ml. of boiling water. It should then be allowed to cool and 60 ml. of this water should be taken every two hours. It stops burning and bleeding in cystitis.

Mango

The mango enjoys a unique status among the fruits of the tropics. It is regarded as a valuable article of diet and a household remedy for several ailments. The ripe mango is antiscorbutic, diuretic, laxative, invigorating, fattening and astringent.

Mango has been found effective in fighting infections. All bacterial invasions are due to poor epithelium. Liberal use of mangoes during the season contributes towards the formation of healthy epithelium, thereby preventing frequent attacks of common infections such as cold, infection, rhinitis and sinusitis. This is attributable to high concentration of vitamin A in mangoes.

The bark of mango tree has also been found especially valuable in diphtheria and other throat infections. Its fluid can be locally applied and also used as a gargle in treating this condition. This gargle is prepared by mixing 10 grams of the fluid extract with 125 ml of water.

Margosa

This tree is very common in India. It has played a key role in Ayurvedic medicine and agriculture since time immemorial. The tree is generally considered to be an air purifier and a preventive against malarial fever and cholera.

An infusion or a decoction of the fresh leaves is a bitter vegetable tonic and alterative, especially in chronic malarial fevers because of its action on the liver. It should be taken in doses of 15 to 60 grams.

Cleaning the teeth regularly with a neem twig prevents gum diseases. It firms up loose teeth, relieves toothache, evacuates the bad odour and protects the mouth from various infections.

Onion

Onion is an exceptionally strong antibiotic and antiseptic food. It was used to treat infections in wounded Russian soldiers during World War II. Latest researches have confirmed the bactericidal properties of onion. According to these findings, if a person consumes one raw onion every day by thorough mastication, he will be protected from a host of tooth disorders. The Russian Doctor, B.P.Tohkin, who has contributed to this research, has expressed the opinion that chewing raw onion for three minutes is sufficient to kill all the germs in the mouth. Placing a small piece of onion on the bad tooth or gum often allays toothache.

Onion can help prevent cholera infection during epidemic. It should be cut into pieces and scattered all over the house during cholera epidemic. This will prevent attack of the diseases. A sauce prepared from onion can also be beneficially used with food during cholera epidemic, this will help prevent the disease. The method of preparing this sauce is to peel the onion and cut it into small pieces. These pieces should then be washed in a small amount of water several times. Vinegar and common salt may be added to taste. This sauce may be used with each meal. It is quite tasteful and effective against cholera.

Another effective onion preparation for preventing cholera is to take 30 grams of onion and seven black peppers. They should be pound in a pestle very finely and then given to the patient of cholera in small doses, two or three times daily. This will allay thirst and restlessness and patient will feel better. It will also reduce vomiting and diarrhoea immediately.

The juice extracted from an onion can be used beneficially to treat pus formation in the ear caused by middle-ear infection. It should be slightly warm and put into the ear two or three times daily.

Pineapple

The pineapple is one of the best fruits of the tropics. It is universally popular fruit, with its distinctive flavour and exquisite taste and above all its refreshing qualities. The fruit is rich in various nutrients.

This popular fruit and its main constituent bromelain, both possess antibacterial activity. It is thus beneficial in the infectious diseases like throat infection, diphtheria and tuberculosis. Fresh pineapple juice exercises a soothing effect on the throat. It is valuable for the singers who often take it for maintaining health of the throat. In diphtheria, it is used as a mouthwash for removing the dead membranes from the throat.

Pineapple juice has proved beneficial in the treatment of tuberculosis. It is found to be effective in dissolving mucus and aiding recovery. This juice was used regularly in the past in treating this disease when it was more common than it is at present. One glass of pineapple juice should be taken daily for this purpose.

Radish

The radish is one of the most commonly used vegetables in India. It has a pungent flavour. It stimulates appetite and promotes a healthy blood stream. The radish is one of the richest sources of iron, calcium and sodium.

This vegetable is valuable in fighting infections. A syrup prepared by mixing a teaspoon of fresh radish juice with equal quantity of honey and a little rock salt is beneficial in the treatment of hoarseness, whooping cough, bronchial disorders and other chest complaints. It should be given thrice daily.

Sage

Sage, one of the most important culinary herbs, has always played a great role in the history of botanic medicine. It is an antibacterial food with antiseptic property. It is especially valuable against infections like sore throat and tonsillitis as well as plague. German doctors commonly recommend a hot sage gargle for sore throat and tonsillitis, says Michael Castleman, author of *The Healing Herbs*. According to him, sage's therapeutic benefit comes from its astringent tannins. This gargle is prepared by putting one to two teaspoons of dried sage leaves in a cup of boiling water. It should be kept steeped for ten minutes. Children under the age of two years, however, should not be given this medicinal dose of sage. Leafy sprigs of sage were spread with brushes on the floors of old manors, as a preventive measure against plague and other infections.

Turmeric

Turmeric is a perennial plant. The rhizomes or underground stems are short and thick and constitute commercial turmeric. It is an important common flavouring spice of daily use. Turmeric has been mentioned in early Sanskrit works and has been used as medicine by the Ayurvedic and Unani practitioners in India since ancient times.

Turmeric is a truly marvelous medicinal spice of the world. It contains antiseptic property and is an effective remedy for cold, rhinitis and throat infection. Half a teaspoon of fresh turmeric powder, mixed in 30 ml. of warm milk, is a useful prescription for treating these conditions. The powder should be put into a hot ladle. Milk should then be poured in it and boiled over a slow fire. In case of running cold, smoke from the burning turmeric should be inhaled. It will increase the discharge from the nose and bring relief. The Paste of fresh turmeric can be applied with beneficial results over skin to cure ringworm, scabies and indolent ulcers.

The juice of raw turmeric is also very effective in the treatment of ringworm infection. It should be applied externally to the parts of the skin affected by ringworm. Simultaneously, one teaspoon of turmeric juice, mixed with an equal quantity of honey, should be taken orally.

CHAPTER 2

ANTI-COAGULANT FOODS

Aspirin, one of the best blood-thinning or anticoagulant medicines, was derived from the bark of a willow tree. It was only in 1970s, that a hormone like substance called prostaglandin was discovered. With this discovery, the scientists began to understand how aspirin works. They now know that the drug has anti-platelet-aggregation powers. It discourages platelets, the smallest blood components, from clumping together or aggregating. They are thus less sticky and less able to build clots that can clog arteries.

This is one of the reasons why doctors believe that low doses of aspirin help ward off heart attacks and strokes. Only 30 mg of aspirin inhibits platelet clumping. Aspirin works by blocking action of a prostaglandin-like substance called thromboxane which otherwise would stimulate platelets to stick together.

With this discovery, scientists began to study other plants and foods, which would also work through the prostaglandin system to inhibit platelets clumping. There are certain food compounds which like the aspirin, are antagonists to thromboxane.

Latest studies suggest that diet can have enormous influence on blood clotting factors. Indeed, evidence suggests that the major influences of diet on heart disease have more to do with blood clotting factors than with blood cholesterol. The benefits of eating to modify blood clot factors are likely to work fairly quickly. A prominent French health official, Dr. Serge C. Renaud, says preventing blood clots can sharply cut your chances of heart attack within a year, whereas it usually takes longer to reduce heart attack risk by lowering cholesterol. However, many foods, such as onions and garlic, do both and so they provide double benefits.

FOODS THAT PREVENT BLOOD CLOTS
Chilli Pepper, Clove, Fruits & vegetables, Garlic, Ginger, Grapes, Mushrooms (Black), Olive Oil and Onion.

Chilli Pepper

Hot chilli peppers are a powerful anti-coagulant food. They are very effective in preventing blood clots. This evidence comes from Thailand, where people eat capsicum chilli peppers as a seasoning and as an appetizer. This infuses their blood with chilli pepper compounds several times a day. Research scientists believe that this may be primary reason why thrombo-embolisms, which is life-threatening blood clots, are rare among Thais.

To prove the theory, hematologist Sukon Visudhi-phan, M.D., and colleagues at the Siriraj Hospital in Bangkok conducted a test. They fortified homemade rice noodles with hot pepper, using two teaspoons of fresh ground capsicum pepper in every 200 grams of noodles. Then they fed the peppery noodles to 16 healthy medical students. Four others ate plain noodles. Almost immediately, the clot-dissolving activity of the blood of the eaters of pepper-laced noodles rose but returned to normal in about 30 minutes. Nothing happened to the blood of the plain noodle eaters.

The effect of chilli pepper was thus short-lived. However, Dr. Visudhiphan believes that frequent stimulation through hot chillies continually clears the blood of clots. This makes Thai people generally less vulnerable to blockage of arteries.

Clove

This popular spice is a powerful anti-coagulant food. It helps keep the blood free of dangerous clots. According to Dr.

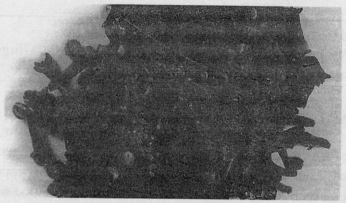

Clove is a powerful anti-coagulant food, which helps keep the blood free of dangerous clots.

Krishna Srivastava of Odense Univerity in Denmark, cloves are stronger than aspirin in this respect. The primary active agent in this spice is eugenol, which also helps protect the structure of platelets even after they have been "aggregated". Dr. Srivastava says that the clove works through the prostaglandin system more or less in the same way as do aspirin, garlic and onion. Cloves help reduce the production of thromboxane, which is a powerful promoter of platelet clumping.

Fruits and Vegetables

Fruits and vegetables high in vitamin C and fibre help prevent blood clots. Those who eat fruits and vegetables in liberal quantities have the most effective clot-dissolving systems, according to a recent Swedish study of 260 middle-aged adults. Those who ate the least fruits and vegetables had the most sluggish clot-dissolving activity. Other research studies indicate that vitamin C and fibre concentrated in fruits and vegetables also improve substantially clot-dissolving mechanisms and help prevent platelet clumping that leads to clots.

Further, the lowest levels of clot-promoting fibrinogen are found in vegetarians. This is especially true in case of vegans who eat no animal products at all, not even eggs and milk. This is presumably due to the fact that compounds in fruits and vegetables lower fibrinogen, while animal fat and cholesterol increase it.

Garlic

Garlic is a powerful anti-coagulant food. It effectively prevents dangerous blood clotting. Even in moderate dietary amounts, it will help thin the blood, thereby reducing its tendency to form blood clots within the arteries. This was discovered by research scientist in the mid-1970s. Studies were conducted in India on Jain religious sect. While some Jains abstain completely from onions and garlic, on religious grounds, others eat them in large amounts. A third group eats a moderate amount. The three population groups are very similar in most other respect, making it easier for a controlled study of garlic and onion. Those Jains who eat garlic and onions liberally, consumed nearly 500 grams of onions and at least 17 garlic cloves in a week. It was found that the blood of these people had less tendency to clot than the blood of the other groups, and the group that did not eat garlic and onion at all had the highest tendency to clot.

Drugs that thin blood are often prescribed after strokes, heart attacks, or blood clots in the legs or lungs. The use of Garlic can interfere and render this drug more potent and as well reduce the side effects from improper doses.

Garlic does not appear to make much difference whether it is taken raw or in cooked form for its blood-thinning effects. A group of researchers studied twenty patients who already had heart disease. The patients took garlic in either raw or fried form for four weeks. Researchers measured their blood fibrinolytic activity, which is a measure of the tendency of the blood to form clots. Within six hours after administration, fibrinolytic activity increased by 72 per cent with raw garlic and by 63 per cent with cooked. These levels remained constant up to twelve hours after administration of a single dose of garlic. The levels rose steadily throughout the next four weeks of the trial, until after twentyeight days the activity with raw garlic was 85 per cent above normal and 72 per cent above normal with cooked garlic.

Ginger

Ginger possesses a strong anti-coagulant property. Blood can be kept free of dangerous clots by eating liberal quantities of this spicy food. It reduces the production of thromboxane. According to Dr. Krishna. C. Srivastava, ginger compounds are strong inhibitors of prostaglandin synthesis than the drug indomethacin, known for its potency.

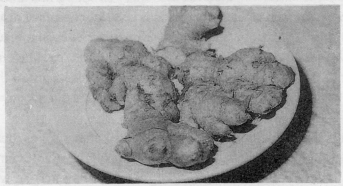

Ginger possesses a strong anti-coagulant property.

Ginger is proven anti-coagulant in humans. This was discovered by Dr. Charles R. Dorso, M.D. of the Cornell University Medical College. He ate large quantity of Crabtree & Evelyn Ginger with Grapefruit Marmalade which was 15 per cent ginger. When his blood did not coagulate as usual, he did a test by mixing some ground ginger with his own blood platelets, and found them less sticky. According to Dr. Dorso the active agent in ginger is gingerol, which chemically resembles aspirin.

Grapes

The grape, known as 'The Queen of Fruits', is one of the most valuable gifts of nature. Charaka, the great physician of ancient India, called it the noblest of all fruits. It has immense therapeutic value, whether eaten as a whole, with skin, pulp and seeds, or used in the form of juice extracted from grapes. This fruit possesses anti-coagulant property and it helps prevent the formation of blood clots. Its skin in particular contains resveratrol, which has been shown to inhibit blood platelet clumping and consequent blood clot formation.

Mushrooms (Black)

The Asian black fungus mushrooms are a valuable food that wards off clots. It is considered a formidable food in Chinese traditional medicine for its beneficial effects on blood. Dr. Dale Hammerschmidt, M.D., a haematologist at the University of Minnesota Medical School, once ate a large quantity of Mapo doufu, a spicy Asian bean curd dish, containing the mushrooms. After eating he noticed dramatic changes in the behavior of his blood platelets. They had much less tendency to clump. He attributed this to anti-coagulant effect of the black mushrooms. The black mushrooms are said to contain several blood-thinning compounds, including adenosine, also present in garlic and compounds, including adenosine, also present in garlic and onions. However button mushrooms do not contain these compounds. Dr. Hammerschmidt concluded that the combination of so many anti-clotting foods in the Chinese diet such as garlic, onions, black mushrooms and ginger may help account for their low rates of coronary artery disease.

Olive Oil

This oil is a potent anti-coagulant food. It retards the stickiness of blood platelets, which may account for its artery protecting powers. This is evident from a research study conducted by British Scientists at the Royal Free Hospital and School of Medicine in London. These researchers made volunteers take three quarters of a tablespoon of Olive oil twice a day for eight weeks in addition to their regular diet. Their platelet clumping was considerably reduced. The scientists found that platelet membranes contained more oleic acid, the dominant fatty acid in olive oil, and less arachidonic fatty acid that encourages stickiness.

The olive-oil-fed blood platelets also released less thromboxane A2, a substance that commands platelets to cling together. Researchers concluded that olive oil benefits platelet function. They believed that this is one more explanation as to the people that depend heavily on olive oil, as in the Mediterranean area, have less heart disease.

Onion

Onions are an anti-coagulant food. Eating them either in raw or cooked form, helps keep blood free of clots. Harvard's Dr. Victor Gurewich advised all his patients with coronary heart disease to eat onions daily, partly because their compounds hinder platelet clumping and increase clot dissolving activity.

In fact, onions have a truly wonderful ability to counteract the detrimental clot-promoting effects of eating fatty foods. This was shown by Dr. N.N. Gupta, professor of medicine at K.G. Medical College in Lucknow. He first fed men a very-high-fat meal, with butter and cream, and discovered that their clot-dissolving activity greatly decreased. Then he gave them the same fatty meal, this time adding 55 grams of onions, raw, boiled or fried. Blood drawn two and four hours after the fatty meal showed that the onions had totally blocked the fat's detrimental blood-clotting proclivities. Infect, 100 grams of onions completely reversed the fat's damaging effects on clot-dissolving activity.

CHAPTER 3

ANTI-DEPRESSANT FOODS

Hippocrates (460-370 B.C.), the father of medicine, included depression in his classification of mental illness. It has been called 'the common cold of psychiatry'. It is the most prevalent of all the emotional disorders. It may vary from feelings of slight sadness to utter misery and dejection. It is the most unpleasant experience a person can endure and is far more difficult to cope with than a physical ailment. It is now firmly established that what one eats has a profound effect on moods. Although food choices may depend on taste or other conscious criteria, there is evidence that people often make unconscious food choices that change brain chemistry and put them in a better mood. These foods serve as anti-depressants. Chronic depression has also been linked to a long-term subtle deficiency of certain nutrients that presumably can go unnoticed and uncorrected by the body for long periods.

Foods seem to manipulate mood by effecting serotonin, one of the brain's most remarkable neurotransmitters. Eating foods that deplete serotonin in the nervous system can make people depressed and their mood bad. On the other hand, taking foods that lead to normal amounts of serotonin in the brain elevates moods more or less in the same way as do the drugs.

FOODS THAT ELEVATES MOODS

Apple, Asparagus Root, Cardamom, Cashewnut, Chilli Pepper, Garlic, Green Vegetables, Honey, Lemon balm, Selenium Rich-Foods and Vitamin B-Rich Foods.

Apple

The apple, a sub-acid fruit, is a highly nutritive food. It contains an abundance of minerals and vitamins. Apples are invaluable in the maintenance of good health and in the treatment of many ailments. The modern saying 'An apple a day keeps the doctor away', sums up the healthful and nourishing qualities of this fruit.

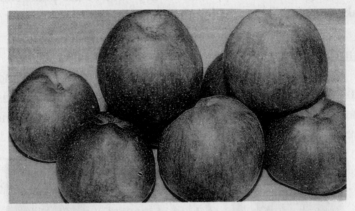

Apple is regarded as an anti-depressant food, which can help overcome mental depression.

This fruit is regarded as an anti-depressant food, which can help overcome mental depression. The various chemical substances contained in this fruit such as vitamin B_1, phosphorous and potassium help the synthesis of glutamic acid, which controls the wear and tear of nerve cells. The fruit should be eaten with milk and honey. This will act as a very effective nerve tonic and recharge the nerves with new energy and life, thereby elevating moods in case of depression.

Asparagus Root

The asparagus is a vegetable of great importance in the diet because of its valuable salts and vitamins as well as for its large amount of cellulose contents. It has been cultivated throughout the temperate zones from the earliest times. It is an alkaline foodstuff, with multipurpose therapeutic properties.

The root of asparagus is an anti-depressant food and helps elevate moods. It makes an effective herbal medicine for the treatment of depression and other mental disorders. It is highly nutritious food and a good tonic for the brain and nerves. One or two grams of the powder of dry root of the plant can be taken once daily in treating these conditions.

Cardamom

Cardamom is one of the most popular spices and is called 'Queen of Spices'. It is one of the most valued spices in the world. The aroma and therapeutic properties of cardamom are due to its volatile oil.

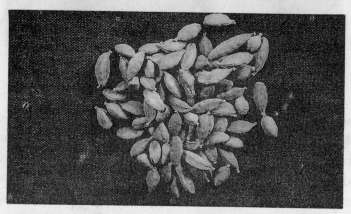

Cardamom is a mood elevating food and a decoction prepared from it can help overcome depression.

This spice is a mood elevating food and a decoction prepared from it has been found valuable in overcoming depression. This decoction is prepared by powdering the seeds and boiling them in water. This decoction should be taken mixed with honey. It has a very pleasant aroma and it helps lift moods in case of depression.

Cashewnut

The cashewnut is a popular nut, which is sweet and very delicious in taste. It is a valuable food both for physical and mental health. It is a complete nourishing diet and a food medicine for several ailments.

The cashewnut is a valuable food for general depression and nervous weakness and it helps elevate moods. It is rich in vitamins of the B group, especially thianmine, and therefore helps stimulate the appetite and the nervous system. It is also rich in riboflavin, which keeps the body active, cheerful, and energetic.

Chilli Pepper

Hot chilli pepper is a mood elevating food and therefore beneficial in the treatment of depression. Its use can give a person a thrill that is more than purely sensory. According to Dr. Paul Rozin, a psychologist at the University of Pennsylvania, who has done extensive research on reactions to hot peppers, the capsaicin, the hot substance contained in it, can induce in the brain a rush of endorphins that can temporarily elevate mood.

Dr. Rozin explains that when a person eats hot chillies, the capsaicin "burns" the nerve endings of the tongue and mouth, causing them to send false pain signals to the brain. In response, the brain tries to protect the body from perceived injury by secreting natural painkillers or endorphins. This gives a lift in the mood and person experiences a sense of well being.

Garlic

The use of garlic helps elevate mood. Many researchers, studying garlic for its effects on blood and cholesterol, noticed that those who ate garlic experienced a definite lift in mood and had a greater feeling of well being. This was especially noted by a German researcher at the University of Hanover. He recently tested a special garlic preparation on people with high cholesterol. The garlic eater, according to questionnaires, felt much better after the garlic therapy. They experienced notably less fatigue, anxiety, sensitivity, agitation and irritability. The power of garlic as mood elevator can be attributed to its richness in selenium and its antioxidant activity.

Green vegetables

Green vegetables are highly beneficial in elevating mood. If a person is suffering from depression, it is possible that he may not be taking sufficient greens like spinach, fenugreek, and green beans in his diet. Medical authorities believes that folic acid or folate deficiency, which is wide-spread, especially among women, can lead to psychiatric disorders, notably depression. Folic acid is a B vitamin, first isolated from green leafy vegetables. It is also heavily concentrated in legumes. Scientists agree that folic acid can act as an anti-depressant. Besides green leafy vegetables, folic acid is found in whole grain cereals and nuts. Dr. Young of McGill University has accumulated considerable evidence to indicate that folic acid deficiency can contribute to depressed mood, and that eliminating the deficiency often cures the condition.

Dr. Young explains how folic acid affects the brain. He notes that patients with various psychiatric disorders, particularly depression, have much higher rates of folic acid deficiency than the general public. Also, psychiatric patients with low folic acid are more severely disturbed. There are good reasons why a lack of this vitamin can cause depression, he says. Folic acid deficiency causes serotonin levels in the brain to fall. In a research study, people deliberately deprived of folic acid, lapsed into sleeplessness, forgetfulness and irritability, after five months. When this vitamin was restored, the symptoms mostly disappear in two days.

Folic acid is needed in very small amounts to fight depression. Dr. young suggests that 200-500 micrograms of folic acid a day may help fight depression in certain susceptible people. That much is easily attainable in food. He, however, cautions that high folic acid dose may be avoided as it may prove toxic.

Honey

Honey is regarded as a mood elevator. It is one of the best remedies for physical and mental tension. Whenever a person feels depressed and tired, he should take two teaspoons of honey dissolved in warm water. This will help overcome depressive mood. Honey contains levulose, dextrose and other sugars, which gives instant energy and a person feels active and stimulated after its ingestion. An excellent brain tonic is to soak seven almonds in water overnight and take them with a tablespoon of honey in the morning after removing the skin.

Lemon Balm

Lemon balm is an important culinary herb of the mint family. It is considered as an anti-depressant food and has been used successfully in the treatment of mental depression. It alleviates brain fatigue, lifts the heart from depression and raises the spirits. A cold infusion of the balm taken freely is reputed to be excellent for its calming influence on the nerves. About 30 grams of the herb should be placed in half a litre of cold water and allowed to stand for twelve hours. The infusion should then be strained and taken in small doses throughout the day.

Selenium-Rich Foods

There is interesting new evidence that eating foods rich in trace mineral selenium can improve moods. Psychologists David Benton and Richard cook, at University College in Swansea, recently discovered that people eating the least selenium were the most anxious, depressed and tired, and generally felt much better when they got adequate selenium.

In a controlled study, 50 healthy men and women, aged 14 to 74, took either 100 micrograms of selenium a day or medicine for five weeks. After six months, they switched to the opposite pill. The selenium in their diet was also measured. Throughout, tests were conducted to judge their moods as to whether they were more composed or anxious, agreeable or hostile, elated or depressed, confident or unsure, energetic or tired and clear-headed or confused. The surprising results were that mood improved markedly when the subjects got enough selenium. Further, the greater their previous selenium deficiency, the greater their lift in mood.

The researchers concluded that a subtle selenium deficiency, not enough to cause the disease, puts a curb on mood. Thus, correcting the slight deficiency would normalize the mood, but getting more of the mineral does not boost mood further. Rich vegetarian sources of selenium are garlic, onions, tomatoes and milk. Selenium influences mood presumably due to its antioxidant power.

Vitamins B-Rich Foods

Vitamin B deficiency has also been associated with depression. Dr. Priscilla, associate clinical professor at the

University of California, prescribes nutritional therapy to build up brain chemicals, such as serotonin and norepine-phrine that affect mood and are often lacking in depressed people. She recommends eating foods rich in B Vitamins, such as whole grains and green vegetables.

CHAPTER 4

ANTI-DIABITIC FOODS

Diabetes mellitus is a nutritional disorder, characterised by an abnormally elevated level of blood glucose and by the excretion of the excess glucose in the urine. It results from an absolute or relative lack of insulin, which leads to abnormalities in carbohydrates metabolism as well as in the metabolism of protein and fat.

In 1550 B.C., the famous Ebers Papyrus advised treating diabetes with high-fibre wheat grains. Not much has changed since then. Plant foods are still the drug of choice for treating diabetes, but now scientists have much more sound reasons for their effectiveness in this disease. Through the centuries, more than 400 plants have been prescribed as remedies for diabetes. Raw onions and garlic have long been favorite anti-diabetic drugs in Europe, Asia and the Middle East. The vegetable bitter gourd and the herb ginseng have been popular drug for diabetes since ancient times in India and China respectively. The common mushroom is widely used in some parts of Europe to lower blood sugar. Barley bread is a popular treatment for diabetes in Iraq. Other foods, which are being used for the treatment of diabetes in various countries, include alfalfa, beans, cabbage, cinnamon, coriander seeds, cucumber, fenugreek seed, Indian gooseberry, Jambul fruit, lettuce and turnips.

All these foods have been shown to possess anti-diabetic property. The tests conducted in modern times have also confirmed that most of these foods or their compounds can lower blood sugar or stimulate insulin production.

Herein are described some of the more important foods which help lower blood sugar or increase insulin production in diabetes patients.

FOODS THAT LOWER BLOOD SUGAR

Artichoke, Bengal Gram, Bitter Gourd, Black Gram, Broccoli, Butea Leaves, Cinnamon, Curry Leaves, Fenugreek Seeds, Fiber-Rich Foods, Foods high in antioxidants, Garlic, Grapefruit, Indian Gooseberry, Isphagula, Jambul Fruit, Kidney Bean Or French Bean, Low-Carbohydrate vegetables, Mango Leaves, Margosa, Onion, Potassium-Rich Foods, Sweet Potato Leaves and Soyabean.

Artichoke

Artichoke, also known as Agathi flower, is a tuberous root with a top like a sunflower. It has a great value as an antidiabetic food. This vegetable contains good amount of potassium, a fair amount of calcium and some iron and sulphur, all of which are needed daily by the body for maintaining good health.

Artichoke is beneficial in the treatment of diabetes because of it's high insulin content. This remedy should however be used by diabetes patient in autumn season, as in this season it is fully ripe and is said to contain more than two per cent of insulin. This insulin is converted into sugars during winter. Artichoke should be eaten raw in salads. If it has to be taken in cooked form, it should be boiled in small amount of water for about 10 minutes. It should not be peeled but cooked whole and may be combined with other vegetables.

Bengal Gram

Bengal gram, also known as chicken pea, is one of the most important pulses in India. It is consumed both in the form of whole dried seeds and in the form of dhal, prepared by splitting the seeds in a mill and separating the husk. Bengal gram has many medicinal properties. Soaked in water overnight and chewed in the morning with honey, the whole gram seed acts as a general tonic. The liquid, obtained by soaking the seeds and then macerating, also serves as a tonic.

Bengal gram is of great value as an anti-diabetic food. Experiments have shown that the oral ingestion of the water extract of Bengal gram increases the utilisation of glucose in both the diabetic and normal persons. Tests were conducted at C.F.T.R.I. Laboratories in Mysore, on a chronic diabetic patient whose insulin requirement was of the order of 40 units a day. When kept on a diet, which included liberal supplements of Bengal gram extract, the condition of the patient improved considerably and his insulin requirement was reduced to about 20 units per day.

Diabetic patients who are on a prescribed diet which does not severely restrict the intake of carbohydrates, but includes liberal amounts of Bengal gram extract, have shown considerable improvement in their fasting blood sugar levels, glucose tolerance, urinary excretion of sugar and general condition.

Bitter Gourd

The bitter gourd is a common vegetable cultivated extensively all over India. It has excellent medicinal virtues. It is antidotal and is useful in reducing fever, strengthening the stomach and promoting its action.

Bitter gourd is specifically used as a folk medicine for diabetes from ancient times in India. Researches by a team of British doctors have established that it contains insulin-like principle, designated as 'plant-insulin', which has been found beneficial in lowering the blood and urine sugar levels.

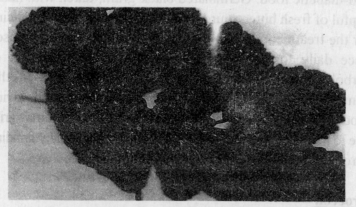

Bitter Gourd has been specifically used as a folk medicine for diabetes from ancient times in India.

This vegetable is thus an effective anti-diabetic food and should be included liberally in the diet of the diabetic. The juice of this vegetable has been found more effective than the fruits. The diabetes patient should take the juice of about three or four fruits every morning on an empty stomach. The seeds of bitter gourd can be powdered and added to regular meals. Diabetics can also use bitter gourd in the form of decoction by boiling the pieces in water or in the form of dry powder, which can be taken mixed with liquid foods.

A majority of diabetics also suffer from malnutrition, as they are usually under-nourished. Bitter gourd, being rich in all the essential vitamins and minerals, especially vitamin A, B1, B2, C and Iron, its regular use prevents many complications associated with diabetes such as hypertension, eye complications, neuritis and defective metabolism of carbohydrates.

Black gram

Black gram is one of the most highly prized pulses of India. It is demulcent and cooling and is a nervine tonic. It is an anti-diabetic food. Germinated black gram, taken with half a cupful of fresh bitter gourd juice, forms an effective medicine for the treatment of mild type of diabetes. It should be used once daily for three or four months with restriction of carbohydrates. Even in severe cases, regular use of this combination, with other precautions, is useful as a health-giving food for the prevention of various compli-cations that may arise due to malnutrition in diabetes patients. Milk prepared by grinding sprouted whole black gram is also good for diabetes.

Broccoli

Broccoli is a close relation of the cauliflower, which has long been popular in Europe. It is the Italian, sprouting, or asparagus broccoli which produces many small, loose, green heads.

These popular vegetables have proved to be an effective anti-diabetic food. It is a rich source of chromium, a trace mineral that seems to lower blood sugar. These trace minerals regulate blood sugar, thereby often reducing medication and insulin needs in diabetes patient. If a person has mild diabetes, chromium may save him from getting the full-fledged disease. If a person's glucose tolerance is borderline, chromium can help control it. Even in cases of low blood sugar, it can raise it to normal level. According to Dr. Richard A. Anderson, Ph.D., at the U.S. Department of Agriculture's Human Nutrition Research Center in Beltsville, Maryland, whatever the blood sugar problem, chromium tends to normalise it. Dr. Anderson believes that increase rate of Type II diabetes is partly due to deficiency of chromium in the diet. He cites some 14 studies done during the 1980s, showing that chromium improved glucose tolerance.

The recommended daily allowance for chromium is 50 to 200 micrograms. Some of the foods rich in chromium, besides broccoli, are whole grain cereals, nuts, mushrooms, rhubarb, bengal gram, kidney beans, soyabean, black gram, betel leaves, bottle gourd, pomegranates and pineapples.

Butea Leaves

Butea, also known as "flame of the forest", is a well-known tree of India. The leaves of this tree are an anti-diabetic food and thus valuable in lowering blood sugar in diabetes. They are useful in glycosuria, which is characterised by the presence of a large amount of glucose in urine. The leaves can be chewed orally or taken in the form of an infusion or decoction.

Cinnamon

The Cinnamon is a popular spice, known to ancient physicians even before 2700 B.C. It is a strong stimulator of insulin activity and thus extremely helpful in the treatment of diabetes.

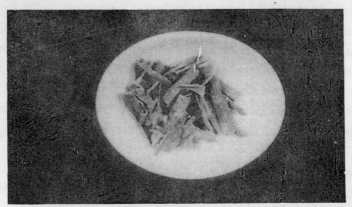

Cinnamon is a strong stimulator of insulin activity and thus useful in diabetes.

Besides cinnamon, there are certain other spices also, which have drug-like property in treating diabetes. They help handle the sugar in sweets to which they are added. Dr. Anderson of United States Drug Administration discovered that some spices help stimulate insulin activity, thereby enabling the body to process sugar more efficiently and thus reducing the need for insulin. He did·some test-tube experiments in which he measured insulin activity in the presence of certain foods. Although most showed no effect, three spices and one herb tripled insulin activity. These are cinnamon, cloves, turmeric and bay leaves. Cinnamon was the most potent.

Only a little cinnamon, such as the small amounts sprinkled on any food item, can stimulate insulin activity, says Dr. Anderson. This will help keep blood sugar in check.

Curry Leaves

Curry leaves, derived from a beautiful, aromatic and more or less deciduous shrub, are slightly bitter and aromatic. They possess the qualities of herbal tonic. They are a food of great value in diabetes.

Eating 10 fresh fully-grown curry leaves every morning for three months is said to prevent diabetes due to hereditary factors. The leaves are also beneficial in the treatment of diabetes resulting from over weight, as they have weight- reducing properties. As the weight drops, the diabetes patients stop passing sugar in urine. The leaves can be taken in form of *chutney* or the juice may be extracted from them and taken in buttermilk or *lassi*.

Fenugreek Seeds

Fenugreek is a well-known leafy vegetable. Its regular use will help keep the body healthy and clean. The leaves of fenugreek are commonly used as cooked vegetable in India.

The seeds of the plant are the best cleansers within the body, highly mucus-solvents and soothing agents.

Fenugreek seeds are a medicine of great value in the treatment of diabetes. According to research studies conducted at National Institute of Nutrition, Hyderabad, fenugreek seeds, when given in varying doses of 25 grams to 100 grams daily diminish reactive hyperglycemia in diabetic patients. Levels of glucose were also significantly reduced in the diabetes patients when the seeds were consumed. These studies indicated that the effect of taking fenugreek seeds could be quite marked, when consumed with 1200 to 1400 calorie diet per day, which is usually recommended for diabetes patients.

Fenugreek seeds can be consumed by diabetics in different ways. A teaspoon of the seeds can be swallowed with water daily. In the alternative, the seeds can be soaked overnight in water and can be taken first thing in the morning. The soaked seeds can also be dried and powdered and this powder taken with milk in doses of one teaspoon twice daily.

Fiber-Rich Foods

The American Diabetes Association had, for decades, recommended low carbohydrate diet for diabetics. In 1979 it realised the error of its recommendations and stated that foods high in dietary fiber should be included in diabetic meals. The British Diabetic Association also recommends high- fiber diet for diabetics.

Foods-rich in fiber are thus considered highly beneficial in the treatment of diabetes. Whole grain cereals are one of the best sources of dietary fiber. A well-known nutritionist, Denis Burkit in his book 'Don't forget fiber in your diet' says "Diabetes decreases and may even disappear in people eating a traditional whole food diet." The British Medical Journal issue dated

December 25, 1979 also supports this view. According to this Journal "A high fiber diet induced a remission of diabetes in 85 per cent of the patients tested." In Britain, between the years 1941 and 1954 it was compulsory to use only high fiber national flour. During that period diabetic mortality rate fell by 54 per cent.

It has been found that the use of soluble fiber contained in barley, oatmeal, fruits, carrots and dried beans, helps considerably in reducing blood sugar levels. The diabetes patients should, therefore, increase gradually such soluble fiber in their diet. High-fibre diets work so well that many patients on such diets have decreased or eliminated their need for supplemental insulin and other anti-diabetic medications.

Foods high in Antioxidants

The diabetes patients should take extra care to have foods rich in antioxidant vitamins E, C and beta-carotene. This advice comes from Dr. James Anderson, M.D., of the University of Kentucky College of Medicine. The reason is that the artery clogging process appears abnormal and more severe in diabetics. The bad-type LDL cholesterol, in diabetics in particular, is more susceptible to oxidation, and thus more likely to become "toxic". In turn, such oxidized LDL is more likely to clog arteries. This may explain two to three times higher risk of heart disease in diabetics, says Dr. Anderson.

The dangerous oxidized cholesterol is caused by high levels of sugar in the blood sustained in diabetes. As sugar is metabolized, it releases the oxygen free radicals that tend to make cholesterol toxic. This can be counteracted by a steady supply of antioxidants.

Main food sources of beta-carotene are carrot, dark orange and dark green leafy vegetables, sweet potatoes, dried apricots, spinach and pumpkins. Vitamin C-rich foods are Indian gooseberry, red and green sweet peppers, broccoli, brussels sprouts, cauliflower, strawberries, spinach, citrus fruits and cabbage. Major food Sources of Vitamin E are vegetable oils, almonds, soybeans and sunflower seeds.

Garlic

Garlic or its constituents have been found in scientific trials to lower blood sugar in diabetes. This vegetable is rich in potassium, which effectively replaces potassium, lost in large quantities in the urine by diabetics. It also contains zinc and sulphur, which are constituents of insulin. Some authorities believe that low levels of zinc may be one of the factors responsible for the onset of diabetes. Garlic also contains manganese, a deficiency of which can contribute towards diabetes.

Garlic has other benefits for diabetics, besides lowering blood sugar. It prevents atherosclerosis, which is a common complication of diabetes. Diabetics can take the equivalent of one or two clove of garlic a day in their diet in any form they liked, such as raw garlic, cooked in food, and capsules. The best way to take garlic, however, is to chew it thoroughly in raw form first thing in the morning.

Grapefruit

The grapefruit occupies a high place among the citrus fruits because of its flavor, its appetising properties and its refreshing qualities. It is an important health-builder and a tonic. It is an anti-diabetic food of great value. Dr. Joe Shelby Riley, a well-known authority on nutrition believes that it is a splendid food for diabetes and if this fruit is eaten more liberally, there would be much less diabetes.

According to him, if a person has sugar, he should use grapefruits three times a day and if a person does not have sugar, but a tendency towards it and wants to prevent it, he should use the fruit three times a day. Simultaneously, he should reduce starches, sweets and fats and eat more fruits and vegetables and juices. In two weeks this will eliminate sugar when not taking insulin. When taking insulin, it takes longer.

Indian Gooseberry

Indian gooseberry is a wonderful fruit and one of the precious gifts of nature to man. It is probably the richest known natural source of antioxidant vitamin C, which is readily assimilated by the human system. It thus contributes greatly towards good health.

Indian gooseberry is an ideal food medicine for diabetes. A tablespoon of its juice, mixed with a cup of fresh bitter gourd juice, taken daily for two months, will stimulate the Islets of Langerhans and enable them to secrete natural insulin. It thus reduces the blood sugar in diabetes. Diet restrictions should be strictly observed while taking this medicine. It will also prevent eye complications in diabetes.

Isphagula

Ispaghula also known as spogel seeds, is an almost stemless small herb covered with dense or soft hairy growth. The medicinal properties of the seeds arise chiefly from the large amount of mucilage and albuminous matter present in them. This herb is an anti-diabetic food and its use has been found beneficial in the treatment of diabetes. It helps control blood sugar in diabetics by inhibiting the excessive absorption of sugars from the intestines.

Isphagula can be taken in the form of seeds or in the form of husk, which is the dry seed-coat of the plant, obtained by crushing the seeds and separating the husk by winnowing. The husk has the same properties as seeds. It has an added advantage that there is no risk of mechanical obstruction or irritation in alimentary canal by the husk. The husk, therefore, is taken without any presoaking and is easier to use than the whole seeds.

Jambul Fruit

The jambul fruit, also known as rose apple or Java plum, is a well-known common fruit, grown all over India. It has been highly appreciated since times immemorial for its unique taste, flavour and colour. This fruit possesses anti-diabetic property. This fruit is regarded in the indigenous system of medicine as a specific treatment against diabetes because of its effect on the pancreas. The fruit, the seeds and fruit juice can all be beneficially used in the treatment of this disease. The 'jamboline' contained in the seeds is believed to have the power to check the pathological conversion of starch into sugar in cases of increased production of glucose. The seeds are dried and powdered. This powder, mixed with water, should be taken three or four times daily. It reduces the quantity of sugar in urine and allays the unquenchable thirst.

In Ayurveda, the inner bark of the jambul tree is also considered valuable in the treatment of diabetes. The bark is dried and burnt. This produces an ash of white colour. This ash should be pestle in the mortar, strained and bottled. The diabetes patient should be given 66 centigrams of this ash on an empty stomach with water in the morning and 1.33 grams each time in the afternoon and the evening, an hour after meals, if the specific gravity of the urine is 1.02 to 1.03. If the specific gravity ranges between 1.035 to 1.055, the ash should be given thrice daily in the quantity of two grams at a time.

Kidney bean or French bean

The beans are one of the most commonly used vegetables all over the world. They have several varieties. The most widespread and widely used bean today is the French bean, also known as common bean or kidney bean.

Beans are high in carbohydrate and fibre. They should be eaten liberally to keep diabetes away and under control. Dr. James Anderson insists that the same foods that lower cholesterol and fight heart disease are excellent also for diabetics, who are at high risk of heart disease. This especially means foods high in soluble fibre like beans. Dr. Anderson says more than 50 studies show that such high-fibre foods significantly reduce blood sugar along with triglycerides and cholesterol.

Kidney or French beans are especially valuable in diabetes. A decoction prepared from this bean is an excellent medicine for diabetes. The procedure is to drink the decoction of French bean pods, one glass every two hours during the day. This decoction is prepared by boiling 60 grams of fresh kidney bean pods, after removal of the seeds, in four litres of water on a slow fire for four hours. It should then be strained through a fine muslin cloth and allowed to stand for eight hours. The decoction must be made fresh every day, as it loses its medicinal value after 24 hours. This treatment should be carried out for four to eight weeks. It is, however, essential to follow strictly the prescribed diet chart.

The juice extracted from French beans is also valuable in diabetes. It stimulates the production of insulin. This juice is generally used in combination with brussels sprout juice in the treatment of diabetes. The patient must, however, be on strictly controlled diet.

Low-carbohydrate vegetables

All vegetables that contain less than three per cent of carbohydrates have been found beneficial in the prevention and control of diabetes. Some of the more important of these vegetables include cucumber, lettuce, radish leaves and spinach. These vegetables should therefore be consumed liberally by the diabetes patients.

Mango Leaves

The tender leaves of the mango tree are an anti-diabetic food. An infusion is prepared from fresh leaves by soaking them overnight and squeezing them well in water in the morning. This filtrate should be taken every morning to control early diabetes. In the alternative, the leaves should be dried in the shade, powdered and preserved for use when necessary. Half a teaspoon of this powder should be taken mixed in water or buttermilk twice a day.

Margosa

This tree is very common in India. It has played a key role in Ayurvedic medicine and agriculture since time immemorial. This tree is generally considered to be an air purifier and a preventive against malarial fever and cholera. All parts of the tree possess medicinal properties. The leaves of this tree are beneficial in the treatment of several common ailments. They also act as an insecticide.

The leaves of Margosa tree possess anti-diabetic property. The use of the juice of these leaves helps in controlling blood sugar in this disease. About five ml. of this juice should be taken early in the morning on an empty stomach for this purpose. This treatment should be continued for three months. In the alternative, 10 leaves should be chewed daily in the morning.

Some communities use dried tender leaves of margosa tree for the prevention and the treatment of diabetes. The leaves should be dried in shade, powdered and preserved in a bottle for use when required. This powder should be taken in small doses of one gram daily.

Onion

Onions have been used as a treatment for diabetes since ancient times. Research studies conducted in Modern times have proved that this pungent vegetable can lower blood sugar in diabetes. In recent investigation in India, Research scientist fed subjects onion juice and whole onions in doses of 25 to 200 grams and found that the greater the dose, the more the blood sugar decrease. It makes no difference whether the onion was eaten in raw or cooked form. The investigators found that the onions affect the liver's metabolism of glucose, or release of insulin, or prevent insulin's destruction.

The probable active hypoglycemic substances in onions are allyl proply disulphide and allicin. In fact, as early as 1923, researchers had detected blood-sugar-lowering property in onion. And in the 1960s, scientist isolated anti-diabetic compounds from onions, which are similar to the common anti-diabetic pharmaceuticals that are used to stimulate insulin synthesis and release.

Potassium-Rich Foods

Foods high in potassium are valuable in diabetes as potassium intake invigorates pancreas. Potassium supple-ments are, however, not beneficial as they may cause ulcer. Diabetics can therefore take foods rich in potassium like raw peanuts, melons, dried peas, potatoes, skimmed milk powder and wheat. Potassium can heal and revitalise the cells of the pancreas, without interference from other food elements.

Sweet Potatoes Leaves

The sweet potato is one of the most nutritious vegetables. It is cultivated all over India for its starchy, pinkish, spindle-like tubers. It is an important source of nutrition in many countries. The leaves of the plant do not have any specific taste and are slightly bitter.

The leaves of sweet potato plant are an anti-diabetic food. They are considered beneficial in lowering blood sugar in diabetes. About 60 grams of fresh leaves or 30 grams of dry leaves along with 100 grams of fresh skin or 12 grams of dry skin of ash gourd should be cut into small pieces and boiled in water. This decoction should be drunk as tea by diabetics with beneficial results.

Soyabean

The soyabean is one of the most nutritious foods. It belongs to the family of legumes or pulses and is perhaps one of the earliest crops cultivated by man. It is esteemed for its high food value. It is a very valuable source of protein, vitamins, minerals and other food ingredients.

Soyabean is a food of great value in the treatment of diabetes. The Journal of the American Medical Association quotes from an authoritative German medical journal, an article by Doctor Christian Becker. In this article, Dr Becker points out that the soyabean is a very valuable food in case of diabetes because bread made from it contains very little starch, but is rich in fat and protein, both of which are of most excellent quality. Soyabean has steadily grown in importance from a therapeutic point of view, since Frieden-wald and Ruhrah showed in 1910 it to be valuable in the feeding of diabetics. Its usefulness in diabetes is attributable not only to its richness in protein and its palatability, but also to its ability to cause, in some unexplained way, a reduction in the percentage and the total quantity of urinary sugar in diabetes patients on the usual dietary restrictions.

CHAPTER 5

ANTI-DIARRHOEAL FOODS

Diarrhoea, commonly known as loose motions, occurs in all human beings periodically from birth to death. Infants and young children are particularly vulnerable to this disease. Most people get the swift attack of this disease for a short duration. For others, it is a habitual and chronic problem with apparently no cause.

The intestine normally gets more than 10 litres of liquid per day. This liquid comes from the diet and from secretions of the stomach, liver, pancreas and intestines. In the case of diarrhoea, water is either not absorbed or is secreted in excess by the organs of the body. It is then sent to the colon where water-holding capacity is limited. Thus the urge to defecate comes quite often.

Diet plays a vital role in controlling diarrhoea. Certain foods counteract diarrhoea effectively as they contain tannins and other astringent compounds. These foods fight bacteria in the intestines and thereby exert a soothing effect. They help drain water out of the gut and solidify faeces. They also help restrict the intestinal track's contractions, which push contents along. In fact, by eating the right food, a person can shorten by one-third to one-half the recovery time from a bout of diarrhoea.

FOODS THAT CONTROL DIARRHOEA

Apple, Babul, Bael Fruit, Banana, Carrot Soup, Chebulic myroblan, Curd, Dill, Drumstick leaves, Fenugreek Seeds, Garlic, Ginger, Guava (unripe), Jambul, Lemon, Mango, Mint, Nutmeg, Pomegranate, Rice, Starchy Fluids and Turmeric.

Apple

Apples are anti-diarrhoeal food. Tissot in 18th century first introduced apple-cure in acute diarrhoea. In recent times, Von-moro and Hessler revived the importance of its curative value in the treatment of this disease. The beneficial effects of the apple-cure are attributed to its pectin and malic acid contents. The pectin swells and engulfs the bacteria that cause diarrhoea and the malic acid inhibits the bacterial growth. In severe types of diarrhoea, supplementing apple juice with specific treatment is found to be very effective.

Grated raw apples have been found especially valuable in infantile diarrhoea. In 1929, Dr. Moro of Heidelberg uses this remedy on a large scale with great success. The method for this treatment is that the child-patient should not undergo any other treatment. Apples, selected from among half-ripe ones, should be peeled, cored and grated. The pulp of the fruit is thus reduced to a soft mass, which rapidly turns brown due to oxidation. The quantity to be used in treating infantile diarrhoea varies between 500 and 1500 grams, depending on the age of the patient. The total quantity to be used should be divided into five meals, varying from 100 to 300 grams at each feeding.

During the first two days of the treatment, child-patient should not be allowed any other food or drink except pure water to quench the thirst so also to prevent dehydration. From third day for two days, he should be given transition diet, which should include only cereals and gruels, and exclude milk and vegetables, before return to the normal diet.

The use of apple juice, mixed with banana, has been found beneficial in the treatment of acute and chronic diarrhoea. Cooked or baked apples are also good for diarrhoea. The cooking process softens the cellulose. Much of its value as a regulating material is thus lost and it is effective in looseness of the bowels.

Babul

Acacia, popularly known as babul tree, is a common large tree, which occurs wild all over India. It is planted for its bark. The tree yields a gum, known as babul gum. The bark of babul tree contains tannin and gallic acid. The leaves and fruits of the tree also contain tannin and gallic acid.

The various parts of this tree are useful in diarrhoea of ordinary intensity. A mixture of equal parts of the tender leaves with white and black cumin seeds can be administered in doses of 12 grams, thrice daily. An infusion made of the bark of the tree may also be taken thrice daily in treating this condition. The gum, used either in decoction or in syrup, is also an effective medicine for diarrhoea.

Bael Fruit

The bael occupies an important place among the indigenous fruits of India. The unripe or half-ripe fruit is perhaps, the most effective anti-diarrhoeal food and is thus valuable food remedy for chronic diarrhoea and dysentery, where there is no fever. Best results are obtained by the use of dried bael or its powder. The bael fruit, when it is still green, is sliced and dried in the sun. The bael slices can also be reduced into powder and preserved in airtight bottles. The unripe bael can be baked and used in such cases with jaggery or brown sugar.

Banana

The banana is one of the oldest and best-known fruits in the world. It is a tropical fruit cultivated all over India. It has a rare combination of energy value, tissue-building elements, protein, vitamins and minerals. The fruit is very hygienic as it comes in a germ-proof package. Its thick covering provides an excellent protection against bacteria and contamination.

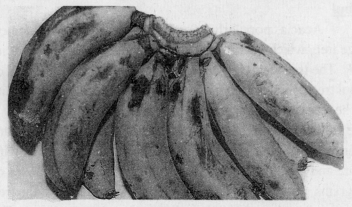

Banana is a powerful anti-diarrhoeal food and it helps control diarrhoea.

Banana is of great value as anti-diarrhoeal food and its use helps control diarrhoea. It normalises colonic functions in the large intestine to absorb large amount of water for proper bowel movements. It also possesses the ability to change the bacteria in the intestines, from the harmful type of bacilli to the beneficial acidophyllus bacilli. It would be advisable to take an exclusive diet of banana, rice and curd during acute stage of the disease.

Carrot Soup

A soup prepared from carrot has been found effective in controlling diarrhoea. It supplies water to combat dehydration, replenishes sodium, potassium, phosphorus, calcium, sulphur and magnesium, supplies pectin and coats the intestine to allay inflammation. It checks the growth of harmful intestinal bacteria and prevents vomiting. Half a kg of carrot may be cooked in 150 ml of water until it is soft. The pulp should be strained and boiled water added to make a litre. Three-quarter tablespoon of salt may be mixed. This soup should be given in small amount to the patient every half an hour.

Chebulic Myroblan

This miraculous herb, known as long-life elixir, has been used in Indian system of medicine for a very long time. The physicians in ancient India used it in the treatment of diarrhoea and dysentery, besides many other elements. It is an effective remedy for chronic diarrhoea and dysentery. Four grams of the pulp of the unripe fruit should be given with honey and aromatics twice a day in the treatment of these diseases.

Curd

Curd or yoghurt is a potent anti-diarrhoeal food of great importance. It is the safest food to prevent and treat diarrhoea, according to tests by Dr. Dennis Savaiano and Michael Levitt of the University of Minnesota. Yoghurt is safe because it is unlikely to harbour bacteria that cause diarrhoea. These two researchers put yoghurt cultures in test tubes with various strains of E.coli bacteria, the number one instigator of traveler's diarrhoea. They found that infection-causing bacteria either died or did not grow. They were, however, found to thrive in ordinary milk.

In another research study at the University of California at Davis, Dr. Georges Halpern found that healthy people who ate 170 grams of ordinary yoghurt a day had a very few bouts of diarrhoea throughout the year. Eating yoghurt may also help recover faster from diarrhoeal infections, according to Dr. Levitt. The bacterial cultures in curd produce lactic acid in the intestine, making the stomach more acidic. This inhibits the ability of infectious bacteria to survive and thrive.

Buttermilk, the residual milk left after the fat has been removed from curd by churning, is also very effective food in diarrhoea. It helps overcome harmful intestinal flora. The acid in the buttermilk also fights germs and bacteria. Buttermilk may be taken with a pinch of salt three or four times a day for controlling this disease.

Dill

The Dill is a green leafy vegetable and a culinary herb. The leaves of this plant are stimulant. They are a soothing and calming medicine and help improve the functional activity of the stomach. The seeds of the plant yield 3 to 3.5 per cent of an essential oil called dill oil, known for its very powerful carminative property.

Dill possesses an anti-diarrhoeal activity. The seeds of this plant, when roasted in ghee with fenugreek seeds in equal quantity, are a specific medicine for diarrhoea and acute bacillary dysentery. For better results, roasted seeds should be powdered and then mixed with curd or buttermilk for use in treating these conditions.

Drumstick Leaves

The drumstick is a fairly common vegetable grown all over India. It is valued mainly for the tender pod. It is anti-bacterial and a wonderful cleanser. Almost all parts of the drumstick tree have therapeutic value. The leaves of this tree possess many medicinal virtues and are therefore beneficial in the treatment of several common ailments. They are full of iron and can be used as food.

The leaves of drumstick tree are an anti-diarrhoeal food. They should be used in the form of juice in controlling diarrhoea. A teaspoon of this juice, mixed with a teaspoon of honey and a glass of tender coconut water, makes a very effective herbal medicine for diarrhoea. It should be given two or three times daily.

Fenugreek seeds

The seeds of fenugreek are a powerful anti-diarrhoeal food. Their use has been found effective in controlling diarrhoea. Half a teaspoon of these seeds should be taken with water three times daily. They have long been used as a folk remedy for diarrhoea in India and Middle East. According to Dr. Krishna C. Srivastava at Odense University in Denmark, this remedy produces quick and marked relief, usually after the second dose.

Garlic

This vegetable is one of the most valuable foods in diarrhoea and other disorders of the digestive system. It aids in elimination of noxious waste matter from the body. As a powerful antibiotic food, it combats bacteria and intestinal parasites. Crushed cloves of garlic may be infused in water and taken to treat this condition.

Ginger

Dry or fresh ginger is highly beneficial in diarrhoea caused by indigestion. A piece of dry ginger should be powdered along with a crystal of rock salt, and a quarter teaspoon of this powder should be taken with a small piece of jaggery. It will bring quick relief, as ginger, being carminative, aids digestion by stimulating the gastrointestinal track.

Guava (unripe)

This fruit is rich in various vitamins and mineral salts, which are essential for the preservation of health and prevention of disease. It is high in food value. The pulp of a ripe guava, mixed with milk and honey, is an excellent natural vitamin C and calcium tonic.

The unripe guava is considered an anti-diarrhoeal food. An infusion of the tender fruit taken with butter-milk is an excellent food for simple diarrhoea, dysentery and sprue. The root-bark is also rich in tannins and can therefore be successfully employed in diarrhoea. It is particularly useful in infantile diarrhoea. A concentrated decoction should be given in treating this condition. This decoction is also administered in cholera for arresting vomiting and diarrhoeaic symptoms.

Jambul

The seeds of jambul are an anti-diarrhoeal food. The

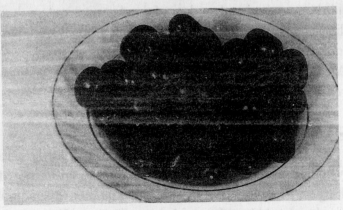

The seeds of Jambul are an anti-diarrhoeal food and an effective medicine for diarrhoea.

powder of these seeds is an effective medicine for diarrhoea. About five to 10 grams of this powder should be taken with buttermilk in treating this condition. The leaves of jambul tree also posses anti-diarrhoeal property. They contain a high concentration of gallic and tannic acid. An infusion of the tender leaves can be taken as a medicine in controlling diarrhoea. This infusion is prepared by soaking 30 to 60 grams of leaves in water. It should be given twice or thrice daily. A decoction of the bark, taken with honey, is also a useful remedy for chronic diarrhoea.

Lemon

Lemon is a powerful anti-diarrhoeal food. It can be beneficially used in controlling diarrhoea. The patient may be given fresh juice of one lemon mixed with 200 ml of water. This process may be repeated several times a day. This treatment can successfully check even the severest type of diarrhoea.

Mango

The juice of this fruit constitutes an anti-diarrhoeal food. It is especially valuable in chronic diarrhoea. For treating this disease, the patient should be given 50 grams of fresh sweet mango juice, mixed with 20 grams of curd and a teaspoon of ginger juice. This may be repeated twice or thrice a day. The quantity of mango juice can be increased from 50 grams to 100 grams, if necessary. This treatment should be continued for a week or so to obtain relief from chronic diarrhoea and dysentery. The leaves of mango tree also form an anti-diarrhoeal food. They contain both gallic and tannic acid and are astringent. A handful of tender leaves should be ground in to a paste or a decoction should be prepared from these leaves and given thrice daily to treat diarrhoea and dysentery.

The use of mango seeds is also valuable in diarrhoea. The seeds should be collected during the mango season, dried in the shade and powdered, and kept stored for use as a medicine, when required. A dose of about one and a half to two gram, with or without honey, should be administered twice daily to treat this condition.

Mint

Mint is a popular spice, used extensively in Indian cooking. It is useful in strengthening the stomach and promoting its action. It also counteracts spasmodic disorders. It forms an ingredient of most drugs prescribed for stomach ailments because of its digestive property.

Mint is an anti-diarrhoeal food. The juice extracted from this plant has been found beneficial in the treatment of diarrhoea. One teaspoon of fresh mint juice, mixed with a teaspoon each of limejuice and honey, can be given thrice daily with excellent results in the treatment of this disease.

Nutmeg

Nutmeg, a popular condiment, is the dried seed or kernel of the fruit, which resembles a small peach and splits when it ripens. It is an anti-diarrhoeal food and its use has been found very effective in controlling diarrhoea. About five to 15 grams of this spice should be powdered and taken, mixed with banana, as a specific medicine in treating this condition.

Pomegranate

The pomegranate is a very delicious and fairly large size fruit, with refreshing and soothing qualities. It possesses anti-diarrhoeal property. It is an astringent food and thus valuable in diarrhoea. In case of weakness caused by profuse and continuous purging, the patient should be given repeatedly about 50 ml of pomegranate juice to drink. This will control diarrhoea. If the patient passes blood with stools, this will stop by the use of fresh pomegranate juice. The flower buds of pomegranate tree are also astringent and are useful in chronic diarrhoea, especially of children.

The rind of the fruit also constitutes an anti-diarrhoeal food. It is astringent and it contains about 28 per cent of tannic acid, identical to gallotannic acid. The rind should be dried and powdered. A decoction should be prepared by boiling 15 to 30 grams of this powder in a glass of water. This decoction can be beneficially used in controlling diarrhoea and dysentery.

Rice

Rice is a much-revered oriental food and the most important tropical cereal. It is the staple food of about half the human race and is often the main source of calories and the principal food for many millions of people.

Rice is one of the safest foods to treat diarrhoea. It has a very low fibre content and therefore soothing to the digestive system. A thick gruel of rice, mixed with a glass of buttermilk and a well-ripe banana, taken twice a day is a very nutritious and ideal diet in diarrhoea.

Starchy fluids

The best remedy for diarrhoea is a starchy fluid. A thick soup or drink made from any starchy food, such as rice, corn, carrot or potatoes, works as medicine in this disease. These foods have long been used in folk medicine as cure for diarrhoea. The most commonly used are rice gruel and carrot soup. Starchy liquids help diminish vomiting, compensate the fluid loss, reduce the duration of the disease and hasten recovery.

Modern research studies have confirmed the efficacy of staple starchy foods. Recently, scientists compared the therapeutic power of such traditional foods with a modern lactose-free infant formula. For instant, in Peru, children suffering from diarrhoea got mixtures of wheat flour or white potato, pea flour, carrots and oil. In Nigeria, they ate a mixture of fermented maize pap, roasted cow pea flour, sugar and palm oil. After the first couple of days, the youngsters on the food mixtures often had less diarrhoea and experienced a return to normal stools earlier than the formula-fed children.

Turmeric

Turmeric is a valuable anti-diarrhoeal food. Its use helps control diarrhoea, especially chronic diarrhoea. This spice is an intestinal antiseptic. It is also a gastric stimulant and tonic. One teaspoon of fresh turmeric rhizome juice or one teaspoon of dry rhizome powder may be taken in a cup of buttermilk or plain water in treating diarrhoea.

CHAPTER 6

ANTI-INFLAMMATORY FOODS

Recent Medical discoveries have shown that foods can reduce inflammation, which is a key process in arthritis and other rheumatic affliction. Leading arthritis specialists now believe that faulty diet may be at the root of these diseases and that correcting it can relieve the symptoms. Studies also show that diet can be a very real aggravator or fighter of these diseases. Scientific studies even support the long prevailing ideas among primitive tribes that certain specific foods may trigger rheumatic diseases and total elimination of those foods will result in a cure.

About 30 years back and before the discovery of hormone-like substances called prostaglandins and leukotrienes, it was difficult to explain how certain foods could possibly influence inflammatory diseases like arthritis and other rheumatic affliction. It is now known that prostaglandins and leukotrienes are manufactured by enzymatic breakdown of a fatty acid called arachidonic acid. What one eats determine how much of the arachidonic acid is present and what type of prostaglandins and leukotrienes—cell messengers that regulate the immune and inflammation process, are created.

Eating a lot of flesh foods and omega-6 type vegetable oils, is likely to create more arachidonic acid, which can set off chain reactions, resulting in specific leukotrienes that cause inflammation. On the other hand, certain foods, such as Garlic and Onion, can manipulate the prostaglandins system to block the process of inflammation. Such foods can intervene in various stages to block the complex biochemical inflammatory process.

FOODS THAT REDUCE INFLAMMATION

Alfalfa, Apple, Castor Seeds, Celery, Cherry, Garlic, Ginger, Grapes, Green vegetable juices, Indian Gooseberry, Lemon, Lemon Grass, Lime, Long pepper, Onion, Pineapple, Potato Juice(raw), Rhubarb, Sesame Seeds, Tamarind, Turmeric, and Vegetables.

Alfalfa

Alfalfa is one of the most nutritionally versatile herbs. It appears to have been discovered by the Arabs who called it the "King of kings" among plants and the "Father of all foods". The seeds, leaves and stems of this plant provide valuable properties for human beings and grazing animals alike. These properties are derived from the plant's ability to penetrate as much as 12 metres into the subsoil so that its roots bring the nourishment of the elusive trace minerals from the depths into the plant's own chemical system.

Alfalfa is an anti-inflammatory food. Its use has been found beneficial in the treatment of arthritis and other inflammatory diseases. A tea prepared from alfalfa, particularly from the seeds, has been found especially valuable. The patients benefit greatly by the alkalizing of food residues aided by alfalfa tea. Six or seven cups of this tea should be taken by arthritis patients for at least two weeks.

The tea from seeds is prepared by cooking them in an enamel pan, with the lid on for half an hour. After cooking, it should be strained, squeezing or pressing seeds dry. It should be allowed to cool and after adding honey to taste put in the refrigerator.

Cold or hot water should be added to taste before use.

Apple

This health-building food possesses anti-inflammatory property. It is regarded as an excellent food medicine for arthritis, gout, and rheumatism, especially when these diseases are caused by uric acid poisoning. The malic acid contained in apple is believed to neutralise the uric acid and afford relief to the sufferers.

The juice extracted from the fruit and an infusion made from the skins is especially valuable in treating these conditions. They have a strong effect against uric acid. These two preparations neutralise an excessive acidity in the blood. Apples, boiled to a jelly, also make a very good liniment for rheumatic pains. They should be rubbed freely on the affected area.

Castor Seeds

The castor is a small annual plant grown as a distinct crop. Castor seeds were an important item of commerce in ancient Egypt. They have been found in tombs dating from 4,000 B.C. In India too, castor has been used since ancient times. In the Susruta Atharvaveda, dating 2,000 B.C., it is referred to as an indigenous and the oil used in lamps. The oil was, and is still, used extensively in medicines.

Though castor plant or its oil is not a food, but still it is one of the most commonly used oils all over the world. It is beneficially used as a safe purgative and as a drug for relieving irritation of the skin and alleviating swelling and pain.

A poultice made from castor seeds can be applied externally to gouty and rheumatic swellings with beneficial results. A decoction prepared from the roots of castor plant with carbonate of potash has also been found very valuable in the treatment of lumbago, rheumatism and sciatica. A paste of the kernel without the embryo, boiled in milk, can also be given as a medicine in the treatment of these conditions.

Celery

Celery is an important salad plant, consisting of the bulbous roots, green leaves and the stem. It has a well-balanced content of basic minerals, vitamins and nutrients, besides a good concentration of plant hormones and essential oils that give celery its strong and characteristic smell.

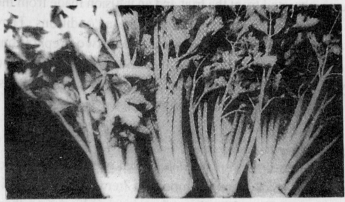

Celery is an anti-inflammatory food and it helps reduce inflammations in arthritis.

This salad plant is an anti-inflammatory food and it helps reduce inflammations in arthritis and other rheumatic affliction. This is attributable to its high sodium content compared with calcium, the ratio being four to one. Its organic sodium tends to prevent and relieve the arthritic joint deposits by keeping lime and magnesia in solution. For best results, it should be taken in the form of freshly extracted juice. Its leaves as well as the stem should be cut into two to five cm pieces before juicing.

Celery is also beneficial in the treatment of rheumatism. A fluid extract of the seeds is more powerful than the raw vegetable.

This also has tonic action on the stomach and kidneys. Five to ten drops of this fluid should be taken in hot water before meals. Powdered seeds can be used as a condiment.

Cherry

Cherry, sweet or sour, is an anti-inflammatory food. It is especially valuable in gout, which is characterised by certain form of inflammation of the joints and swellings of a recurrent type. This was discovered by Lodwig W. Blan, Ph.D., some 50 years back. Himself a gout sufferer, he found the use of cherries to be miraculously effective in his own case and published his own experience in a medical journal. Subsequently, many people with gout used this simple therapy with great success. To start with, the patient should consume about 15 to 25 cherries a day. Thereafter, about 10 cherries a day will keep the ailment under control. While fresh cherries are the best, canned cherries can also be used with success.

Garlic

Garlic possesses anti-inflammatory property. It is known to affect prostaglandin that helps reduce inflammation. Physicians in India noticed during a study of garlic's impact on heart disease that garlic eaters often got relief from joints pain, in particular those with osteoarthritis, which also involves inflammation. During the test, subjects ate two or three raw or cooked garlic cloves every day.

In Russia, garlic is used extensively in the treatment of rheumatism and associated diseases. In Britain also, garlic is recommended to rheumatic sufferers. Recent experiments in Japan tested a garlic extract on patients with lumbago and arthritis and a large number were benefited, without any undesirable side effects.

Garlic is also one of the most effective food medicines in sciatica. It can be used in the form of either raw garlic or garlic milk. In case of raw garlic, it should be cut into small pieces and taken with a teaspoon of honey with each meal. Garlic milk can be prepared both in cooked and uncooked states. Raw uncooked form is more powerful. The milk is prepared by adding the pulp of crushed garlic in uncooked buffalo milk. The proportion is four cloves to 110 ml of milk. In cooked state, it should be boiled in milk. The most popular method is to take the garlic cloves internally, although some reports indicate that pain can also be relieved by rubbing the affected parts with cloves of cut garlic. Garlic oil is rapidly absorbed through the skin and into the bloodstream, and quickly reaches the affected areas.

Ginger

Ginger is a powerful anti-inflammatory drug. It has been used for centuries in Ayurvedic system of medicine to treat various rheumatic and musculoskeletal diseases. In a recent study, Dr. Krishna C. Srivastava of Odense University in Denmark, tested ginger in small doses daily on a group of arthritis patients for three months. Most of them reported less pain, swelling and morning stiffness and more mobility. Dr. Srivastava, who has successfully treated several arthritis patients with ginger, recommends an intake of 5 grams of fresh ginger or half a gram ground ginger three times a day. The ground ginger should be taken after dissolving in a liquid food. The experts opine that ginger seems to have no side effects. In fact, ginger is considered to be superior to the widely prescribed anti-arthritis drugs known as NSAIDs (non-steroidal anti-inflammatory drugs), according to Dr. Srivastva.

Ginger presumably works in two or even more ways. It blocks formation of both prostaglandins and other inflammatory substances called leukotrienes. Further, Dr. Srivastava suggests that ginger's antioxidant activity breaks down inflammatory acids in the joints' synovial fluid.

Dr. Srivastava has also found powdered dry ginger effective in combating pain and swelling from the inflammation of osteoarthritis.

Grapes

Grapes are a valuable anti-inflammatory food. They help reduce inflammation due to their richness in alkaline elements, which tend to dissolve the uric acid. Their use is therefore highly beneficial in the treatment of arthritis, gout and rheumatism. Doctor Tabanera, who has had vast experience in treating patients with grape diet, affirms in the Median Journal Viva Cien Anos that chronic rheumatism and gout can be alleviated by an exclusive diet of grapes and their juices.

Green Vegetable Juices

Green vegetable juices possess anti-inflammatory properties. They help greatly in relieving arthritis and other rheumatic conditions. Green juice extracted from any green leafy vegetable, mixed with carrot, celery and red beet juice, is a specific remedy for these conditions. The alkaline action of raw juices dissolves the accumulation of deposits around the joints and in other tissues, thereby relieving pain and swelling.

Indian Gooseberry

This fruit is of great value as an anti-inflammatory food. Its use has been found beneficial in reducing inflammation in arthritis and other rheumatic conditions. The fruit should be dried in shade and powdered. One teaspoon of this powder,

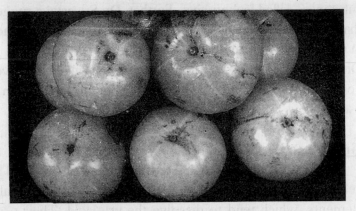

The use of Indian Gooseberry has been found beneficial
in reducing inflammation in arthritis.

mixed with two teaspoons of jaggery, should be taken twice
daily for a month in the treatment of these conditions.

Lemon

Lemon is an anti-inflammatory food. Though the lemon
juice is acid in taste, its reaction in the body is alkaline. Hence,
it is valuable in the treatment of rheumatic affections such as
arthritis, gout, rheumatism, sciatica, lumbago, and pain in hip
joints, which result from too much acid in the body. A sufficient
intake of lemon juice prevents the deposit of uric acid in the
tissues and thus reduces the possibility of an attack of gout and
other rheumatic diseases. In the treatment of rheumatism and
gout through the use of lemon, the patient should begin with one
lemon per day and gradually increase the quantity until he takes
a dozen or more. Thereafter the quantity should be reduced in
the same order until one lemon is taken per day.

Lemon Grass

Lemon grass is a perennial, aromatic tall grass, with

rhizomes and fibrous roots. It is stimulant, tonic, aromatic, antispasmodic and a mild counter-irritant. The oil distilled from its leaves is used for medicinal purposes.

The grass possesses anti-inflammatory property and can thus be beneficially used in the treatment of arthritis and rheumatism. Lemon grass oil mixed with twice its bulk of coconut oil, is a stimulating ointment for rheumatism, lumbago, neuralgia, sprains and other painful affections. In chronic cases, the undiluted oil may be used for better results. It can also be taken internally in the form of raw juice or decoction yielding beneficial results.

Lime

This citrus fruit is an anti-inflammatory food of great importance. It has been used as an effective remedy in arthritis and gout since long. Vitamin C, contained in it, is known to prevent and cure sore joints by strengthening the connective tissue of the body. The citric acid found in the lime is a solvent of uric acid, which are the primary cause of arthritis, gout and other diseases of this nature. It can be taken in the form of juice extracted from the fruit in a glass of warm water, to which a teaspoon of honey may be added. It can be taken twice daily in treating these conditions.

The use of lime is also highly beneficial in the prevention and treatment of inflammation of the gum margins, pyorrhea and dental caries. In a research study, 450 patients with these conditions were given half a lime and 240 ml of orange juice twice a day. This led to the disappearance of most of the inflammation and an arrest of about 50 per cent of caries, besides stimulating body growth.

Long Pepper

Long pepper is a small, slender aromatic plant, having

perennial woody roots with thin and erect branches. It is indigenous to India and is cultivated extensively in many places of Tamil Nadu, West Bengal and Assam. The fruits, the root and thicker parts of stem are cut and dried and used as an important drug in Ayurvedic and Unani medicines.

Long pepper is an anti-inflammatory food. Its use has been found beneficial in the treatment of rheumatic diseases like rheumatism and gout. It should be given in doses of three to five decigrams, mixed with honey. Besides taking internally, it can also be applied locally. It will help relieve muscular pains and inflammation.

Onion

Onion possesses anti-inflammatory activity. Its regular use, especially in raw form, can help reduce inflammation in arthritis and other rheumatic diseases. The juice of this vegetable, mixed with mustard oil in equal quantity, can also be applied externally, with beneficial results, to allay pains and swellings in rheumatic afflictions.

Pineapple

This fruit is an anti-inflammatory food. It helps suppress inflammation. Both the fruit and its main constituent, an antibacterial enzyme called bromelain, are anti-inflammatory. The use of this fruit has thus been found valuable in preventing arthritis and other rheumatic afflictions. Fresh pineapple juice reduces swelling and inflammation both in osteoarthitis and rheumatoid arthritis. An exclusive diet of fresh pineapple juice for few days, and repeated at regular intervals, will help greatly in relieving symptoms of these diseases.

Potato Juice (raw)

The potato is the most popular and widely-used vegetable in the world. It is one of the most strongly alkaline of all foods, being rich in potash and soda. It is therefore, very helpful in maintaining the alkali reserve of the body and a natural antidote for an overdose of acid. It dissolves away uric acid and lime.

The raw potato juice therapy is considered one of the most successful biological treatments for arthritic and rheumatic conditions. It has been used in folk medicine for centuries. The old method of preparing potato juice was to cut the potato into thin slices without peeling the skin and place them overnight in a large glass filled with cold water. The water should be drunk in the morning on an empty stomach. Fresh juice can also be extracted from potatoes and drunk diluted with water on 50:50 basis, first thing in the morning.

Rhubarb

Rhubarb is a vegetable grown for its long thick leaf stalks, which are used for sauces and pies. The dried rhizomes of the plant constitute the drug. The rhizomes should be collected from six or seven years old plants, just before the flowering season. They should not be decorticated. The tuber is pungent and bitter.

Rhubarb is an anti-inflammatory food. It is especially beneficial in the treatment of rheumatism. The green stalks of this vegetable should be pounded with an equal quantity of jaggery. A teaspoonful should be taken three or four times a day. This will alleviate pain and swelling.

Sesame Seeds

The sesame is a well-known oilseed. It is probably the

oldest of all cultivated seed crops. It has been regarded as a food of high value throughout Asia since ancient times. There are three varieties of sesame seeds: black, white and red. The black variety yields the best quality of oil and is also the best to use for remedial purposes. The oil extracted from sesame seeds is of a very high medicinal value.

Black Sesame seeds possess anti-inflammatory property. Their use has thus been found beneficial in the prevention and treatment of frequent joint pains in arthritis and other rheumatic afflictions. A teaspoon of the seeds should be soaked overnight in a quarter cup of water and taken first thing in the morning for this purpose. The water in which seeds are soaked should also be taken along with the seeds.

Tamarind

Tamarind is a large, handsome, symmetrical spreading tree. All the parts of the tree have medicinal virtues. Its leaves are cooling and antibilious, while the bark is an astringent and tonic. The fruit pulp is digestive, antiflatulent, cooling, laxative and antiseptic. Its seeds are also astringent.

The leaves of this tree are an anti-inflammatory medicine and thus highly beneficial in prevention and treatment of arthritis, rheumatism and gout. The leaves should be crushed with water and made into a poultice. This poultice can be applied externally over the inflamed joints and ankles. This will reduce swelling and pain.

Turmeric

This unique medicinal spice is a potent anti-inflammatory food. The active ingredient of turmeric is curcumin, which gives it its intense cadmium yellow colour. Studies show that curcumin is an anti-inflammatory agent on par with cortisone. It has been found to reduce inflammation in animals and symptoms of rheumatoid arthritis in humans. In an experiment, the prime compound in turmeric, improved morning stiffness, walking time and joint swelling in 18 patients with rheumatoid arthritis. In fact, 1,200 mg of curcumin had the same anti-arthritis activity as 300 mg of the anti-inflammatory drug phenylbutazone.

Vegetables

The treatment of arthritis through liberal use of vegetables has been found very effective. Giving up flesh foods may help cure arthritis. This has become evident from a widely acclaimed study conducted in 1991 by Norwegian researchers. This study showed that meatless diets relieved rheumatoid arthritis symptoms in nine out of ten patients. This was because animal fat incites joint inflammation, according to researchers.

Dr. Jens Kjeldsen-Kragh, M.D., of the Institute of Immunology and Rheumatology at the National Rheumatism Hospital of Oslo, conducted a study about the usefulness of vegetarian foods in arthritis. He found that switching to a vegetarian diet resulted in improved grip strength and much less pain, joint swelling, tenderness and morning stiffness in about 90 per cent of a group of arthrites patients, compared with controls eating an ordinary diet. The patients noticed improvement within a month, and it lasted throughout the entire year-long experiment. Dr. Kjeldsen Kragh concluded that about 70 per cent of the patients improved because they avoided fats that are likely to instigate the inflammation process. This proves that vegetable cure is stronger than drugs.

CHAPTER 7

ANTIOXIDANT FOODS

Many of our health problems are due to the perversity of oxygen. The toxic forms of oxygen constantly torment the cells of the body. Oxidants occur in various forms. The most harmful and best-studied are so-called oxygen free radicals. These molecules are charged up and cause trouble. They have lost one of the electrons that keep them chemically stable. In their frenetic search for another one, they will try to grab it from anywhere. They thus destroy healthy cells in this search and create still more groups of free radicals in split-second reactions that become out-of-control chain reactions.

Oxygen free radicals can attack DNA, the genetic material of cells, causing them to mutate, which is a first step towards development of cancer. Perhaps even more frightening: free radicals attack the fatty parts of cell membranes. Left defenseless without enough antioxidants, these fatty molecules become peroxidized or rancid. This can completely disrupt the cell membrane's structure.

Oxidation of fat occurs throughout the body, especially in the cell membranes. Oxidation is opposed by natural system within the body, and antioxidant substances eaten in the diet support it. Antioxidant vitamins, such as vitamins C and E, beta-carotene, and the mineral selenium are all important dietary antioxidants, and diets high in these help prevent atherosclerosis. Anti-dietary oxidants can prevent several damaging effects of oxidants on health. Continual attacks by oxygen reactions can clog arteries, turn cells cancerous, make joints inflamed and nervous system weak. So far, scientists have linked adverse oxygen reactions to at least 60 different chronic diseases. Antioxidants also play an important role in delaying ageing process. Steady supply of antioxidants to the cells protects health and prolongs life more than anything else. Food antioxidants are numerous chemical substances, which fight against oxygen-charged molecules that damage cells. They help prevent most of the chronic diseases like heart disease, cancer, bronchitis and cataracts.

FOODS THAT PREVENT OXYGEN DAMAGE

Asparagus, Broccoli, Brussel sprouts, Cabbage, Carrot, Fruits & Vegetable, Garlic, Ginger, Grapes, Indian Gooseberry, Indoles-Rich Foods, Lettuce, Liquorice, Oats, Onion, Orange, Peanut, Pumpkin, Spinach, Sweet Potato, Tomato, Vitamin E-Rich Foods and Watermelon.

Asparagus

This vegetable is a super source of glutathione, which is a powerful antioxidant compound, strong anticancer activity. The liberal use of asparagus can thus prevents having damage to cells by oxygen-charged molecules. It is good to eat this vegetable raw and mixed with a vegetable salad. If it has to be taken in cooked form, it should be cooked very slightly so as to preserve most of the rich minerals and vitamins contained in the raw vegetable.

According to Dean P. Jones, Ph.D., associate professor of biochemistry at Emory University School of Medicine, glutathione can deactivate at least thirty cancer-causing substances. This compound prevents lipid peroxidation and acts as an enzyme to deactivate free radicals. Thus, it offers powerful protection against heart disease, cataracts and asthma, so also cancer and other diseases linked to free-radical damage. Glutathione also helps prevent damage from toxic compounds such as environmental pollutants by detoxifying them in the body.

Main food sources of Glutathione are avocado and watermelon, besides asparagus. These three foods contain the most glutathione, according to an analysis of 98 popular foods by Dr. Jones. Other foods high in glutathione are fresh grapefruit orange, strawberries, fresh peach, lady finger, white potato, cauliflower, broccoli and raw tomato.

Broccoli

Broccoli is a versatile disease-fighting food. It contains numerous strong antioxidants like quercetin, gluta—thione, beta-carotene, indoles, vitamin C, lutein, glucarate and sulphoraphane. This vegetable possesses extremely high anticancer property, particularly against lung, colon and breast cancers. Like other cruciferous vegetables, it speeds up removal of oestrogen from the body, thereby helping suppress breast cancer. It is rich in cholesterol-reducing fibre and also possesses antiviral and anti-ulcer activities. This vegetable is thus a powerful antioxidant food, which helps prevent several damaging effects of oxidants on health.

Cooking this vegetable destroys some of the antioxidants and anti-oestrogenic agents, such as indoles and glutathione. It is, therefore, advisable to eat it either raw in salad or lightly cooked, preferably steamed. Care should be taken to chew it thoroughly. Unsalted butter or vegetable oil may be used as a dressing.

Brussel sprouts

Brussel. sprouts is one of the distinct vegetables

developed from the original wild cabbage. It may be distinguished when the plants are mature by the sprouts, which are little compact round heads, borne along the erect stem among the leaves. It is rich in Vitamins A, B_1 and C as well as in potassium. Like other cruciferous vegetables, brussel sprouts possess almost the same properties as broccoli and cabbage. It is an anticancer, oestrogenic and contains various antioxidant compounds including indoles. This vegetable is thus an important dietary antioxidant. It helps prevent damage to cells by free radicals.

Brussel sprouts are good to eat chopped and mixed in a salad, or cooked very lightly for about three minutes. Unsalted butter or a vegetable oil may be used as a dressing.

Cabbage

This popular vegetable was revered in ancient Rome as a cancer cure. It contains numerous anti-cancer and antioxidant compounds. It speeds up oestrogen metabolism, thereby helping prevent breast cancer and suppress growth of polyps, a prelude to colon cancer. In studies, eating cabbage more than once a

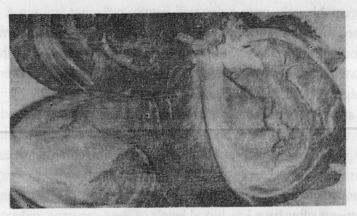

Cabbage contains numerous anti-cancer and antioxidant compounds.

week cut men's colon cancer odds 66 per cent. As little as two tablespoons daily of cooked cabbage is said to protect against stomach cancer. This vegetable also contains anti-ulcer compounds and cabbage juice helps heal ulcers in humans. Cabbage is one of the major food sources of indoles, which successfully detoxify several cancer-causing agents.

Cabbage should be rarely cooked, since it rapidly loses its value through the process even when done conservatively. Cooking also destroys some antioxidant, anti-cancer and oestrogenic activity of compounds, particularly indoles. It is delicious when included in a vegetable salad. It must be masticated thoroughly, raw or cooked, and never swallowed in a hurry.

Carrot

Carrot is an extremely rich food source of beta-carotene. The name carotene, which is a form of pro-vitamin, has been derived from carrot. The carotene is converted into vitamin A by the liver and it is also stored in the organ. Carrot contains so much beta-carotene that liberal intake of this vegetable only, once a day will supply sufficient vitamin A for meeting the requirement of a day. If carrot is to be taken in cooked form, the cooking time should not exceed fifteen to twenty minutes. It can also be baked like potatoes. Butter or vegetable oil may be used for dressing.

Carrot is a strong antioxidant and a powerful cleansing food by virtue of its richness in beta-carotene. Beta-carotene is an orange pigment that helps prevent heart attacks, irregular heartbeats, strokes and cancer, especially lung cancer. It boosts immune functioning and destroys single oxygen-type free radicals. Cancer patients often have low blood levels of Beta-carotene, indicating low beta-carotene in their diets. According to one study, beta-carotene levels in the blood of lung cancer patients was one-third lower than that in healthy individuals.

Other rich food sources, of beta-carotene besides carrot, are dark orange and dark green leafy vegetables, sweet potatoes, dried apricots, spinach and pumpkins.

Fruits & Vegetables

Foods like fresh fruits and vegetables contain a variety of strong antioxidants. They are especially concentrated in quercetin, which is one of the strongest biologically active members of the flavonoid family and a powerful antioxidant. This compound helps prevent several diseases. "Quercetin is one of the most powerful anti-cancer agents ever discovered," says Dr. Terrance Leighton, Ph.D., professor of biochemistry and molecular biology at the University of California at Berkeley. It inactivates several cancer-causing agents, preventing damage to cell DNA, and inhibits enzymes that help tumour growth. Quercetin is also anti-inflammatory, anti-bacterial, anti-fungal and antiviral.

Quercetin is antithrombotic, and thus helps prevent formation of blood clots. As an antioxidant, it absorbs oxygen free radicals and helps keep fat from becoming oxidized. Thus, quercetin helps prevent artery damage from oxygen free radicals and oxidized LDL cholesterol, thereby helps keep arteries clean and open.

When a person eats the antioxidants, as contained in fresh fruits and vegetables, they are infused in the tissue and fluids. There they help resist the attack of oxidants, there by preventing their damaging effects on health. A person can get the most disease fighting antioxidants by liberal intake of raw uncooked fruits especially the deep coloured ones, and fresh raw vegetables.

Garlic

Garlic is a powerful antioxidant. This explains some of its beneficial properties in preventing atherosclerosis, cancer and some other chronic diseases. The garlic constituents that reduce the oxidation of fats in the body are alliin, diallyl heptasulfide, diallyl hexasulfide, diallyl pentasulfide, diallyl tetrasulfide, diallyl trisulfide, S-allyl cysteine, S-allyl mercapto cysteine and selenium.

One clove of garlic has about the same antioxidant power in a laboratory dish as 15 mg of vitamin C or 4.5 mg of vitamin E. Both these doses are low compared to the minimum daily-recommended intake for these vitamins, but garlic may also increase antioxidation in the body by supporting the body's natural antioxidant system and making fats harder to oxidize. Garlic can be used as flavouring in the preparation of cooked food or rubbed after crushing over a salad bowl. However, for best results, it should be chewed raw to derive maximum benefits from its compounds. Excessive use of garlic should, however, be avoided.

Ginger

Ginger has been used for centuries in Asia in treating a variety of diseases. It is more effective in some respect than many costly drugs. Ginger is a powerful antioxidant. It helps prevent and treat migraine and arthritis and acts as an antithrombotic and anti-inflammatory agent in humans. It is an antibiotic in test tubes and anti-ulcer agent in animals. It also ranks very high in anticancer activity.

Ginger is available in two forms, fresh and dried. Both the forms are effective. As the taste of ginger is not very good, it is mostly used in cooked vegetables. It is a common constituent of curry powder.

Grapes

Grapes are rich storehouse of antioxidant and anti-cancer compounds. Red grapes are high in antioxidant quercetin, which is lacking in white and green varieties. The skins of this fruit contain resveratrol that inhibit blood platelet clumping and the resultant blood clot formation. It boosts good-type HDL Cholesterol. Red grapes have shown anti-bacterial and antiviral activities in test tubes. Grapeseed oil also raises good-type HDL Cholesterol.

Indian Gooseberry

Indian gooseberry is a super food source of antioxidant vitamin C. Repe..ted laboratory tests at Coonoor show that every 100 grams of this fresh fruit provides 470 to 680 mgs of vitamin C. A versatile and powerful anti-oxidant, vitamin C seem to protect against asthma, bronchitis, cataract, heart arrhythmias, angina and cancer of all types. It has also stopped the growth of the AIDS virus in test tubes. Many experts believe that the ability of Vitamin C as an antioxidant helps keep LDL cholesterol from becoming oxidized, making it a strong deterrent to clogged arteries and cardiovascular disease. Vitamin C and Vitamin E work together to revitalize and replenish each other.

Main food sources of Vitamin C, besides Indian gooseberry, are red and green sweet peppers, broccoli, brussels sprouts, cauliflower, strawberries, spinach, citrus fruits and cabbage.

Indoles Rich Foods

Indoles are antioxidant compounds. They are one of the earliest classes of anticancer food compounds discovered. They are highly successful in blocking cancer in animals. They work by deactivating cancer-causing agents. In humans, indoles are

especially likely to help prevent colon and breast cancer.
The main food sources of Indoles are cruciferous vegetables like broccoli, brussels sprouts, cabbage and cauliflower, watercress, drumstick, mustard, radish and turnip. Studies at the University of Manitoba found that boiled cruciferous vegetables lost about half of their indoles in cooking water. They should therefore be preferably taken in raw form.

Lettuce

Lettuce is the most popular of all the salad vegetables and is regarded as the king of salad plants. It is a live food with its rich vitamin and mineral content, especially the antioxidant vitamin C. This vegetable is bulky, low in food value but high in health value. It is rich in mineral salts with the alkaline elements greatly predominating. So it helps keep the blood clean, the mind alert and body in good health.

Lettuce is a powerful antioxidant and contains many different antioxidants, including beta-carotene and folic acid, as well as lutein, an antioxidant that some scientists considered as potent as beta-carotene in fighting cancer. Lettuce exhibits extraordinary anti-cancer powers. According to Frederick Khachik, Ph.D., a research scientist at the Department of Agriculture, lutein and other carotenoids are not lost during cooking or freezing, although heat does harm more fragile antioxidants, including Vitamin C and Glutathione.

Liquorice

Liquorice is a popular flavouring agent. It plays an important part in Indian medicine and is one of the principal drugs of the 'Susruta'. It was also frequently used in ancient Egypt, Greece and Rome. It has been known in pharmacy for thousands of years. In old Chinese pharmacy, it was considered to be a first class drug and rejuvenating property was ascribed to it

Liquorice possesses antioxidant property and is a powerful multi-faceted medicine. It also has strong anti-cancer powers, presumably due to high concentration of glycyrrhizin. Experiments have shown that mice drinking glycyrrhizin dissolved in water have a very few skin cancers. This spice also kills bacteria, fights ulcers and diarrhoea.

Liquorice can be chewed or sucked or it can be taken in the form of powder mixed with honey or powdered jaggery. It can also be taken in the form of decoction or an infusion.

Oats

Oats are used for human consumption in the form of oatmeal and rolled oats. A dish of oatmeal, with milk and a little honey, is regarded as a perfect breakfast. It is a pleasant food and is enjoyed by children and old people alike.

Oats possess antioxidant and oestrogenic properties. It helps stabilize blood sugar. A couple of bowls of oat bran or three bowls of oatmeal a day can lower cholesterol 10 per cent or more, depending on individual responses. Oats also contain psychoactive compounds that may combat nicotine cravings and have antidepressant powers. Excessive use of oats should, however, be avoided as their excessive intake can cause gas, abdominal bloating and pain in some persons. Oats, like other cereals, can also trigger food intolerances in susceptible persons and may cause chronic bowel distress.

Onion

Onion is an exceptionally strong antioxidant food. It is one of civilization's oldest medicines. It contains several anticancer compounds. This vegetable is the richest dietary source of quercetin, a powerful antioxidant. This substance is found only in shallots, yellow and red onions and not in white. Some onions are so full of quercetin that the compound accounts for up to 10 per cent of their dry weight, according to tests by Terrance Leighton, Ph.D., professor of biochemistry and molecular biology at the University of California at Berkeley. Onions have been specifically linked to inhibit human stomach cancer. It thins the blood, lowers cholesterol, raises good-type HDL cholesterol, wards off blood clots, and fights asthma, chronic bronchitis, hay fever, diabetes, atherosclerosis and infections. It is considered to possess diverse anticancer powers. Excessive use of onions should, however, be avoided as it may promote gas formation and aggravate heartburn. Recent experiments have also found that abundant use of onions have a tendency to reduce the number of red cells and to lower the haemoglobin.

Orange

The orange is the most popular and widespread of the citrus fruit. It is a very delicious and nourishing fruit. It is a rich source of protective food ingredients like vitamins A, B, C as well as calcium, and its health-promoting properties emanate from these nutrients. Being a predigested food, it produces heat and energy in the body immediately after its use.

Orange is a powerful anti-oxidant food, being rich in antioxidant vitamin C and beta-carotene. It contains all classes of known natural cancer inhibitor, namely carotenoids, terpenes and flavonoids. It protects against several types of cancers, especially pancreatic cancer. By virtue of its richness in Vitamin C, it may ward off asthma attacks, bronchitis, atherosclerosis and gum disease. It may also boost fertility and healthy sperms in some men.

team it in its own juice.

e spinach is a leafy vegetable, with broad green leaves.

e spinach is a leafy vegetable, with broad green leaves.
n among all green vegetables. The leaves are cooling
ritive. They contribute roughage, colour and bland
e diet.

the list of green leafy vegetables, which helps
r. It is an extremely rich source of antioxidants
compounds. It contains about four times more
d three times more lutein than broccoli. This
rich in fibre that helps lower blood cholesterol.
xidants are destroyed in cooking. It should
in raw form or lightly cooked. Spinach is
xalate. Its use should therefore be avoided
from kidney stones.

ritious vegetable is a super food source
otene. According to US department of
ams of mashed sweet potatoes contains
carotene, or approximately 23,000
ral use of this vegetable helps prevent
rokes and numerous cancers.

antioxidant, as a major source of
s it its colour. Lycopene intervene
xygen free radical molecules
ancer agent. For instance, J
opene severely lacking i
cancer. They also ob

Peanut

The peanut, also known as g
bean family and is a legu
because of its high nutriti
family meals and snacks
Peanuts are an extrem
ubiquinol-10. This li
best antioxidants t
found in high cor
be the most eff
vitamin E, in
oxidation, sa
10 also he
Eating fr
very nu
nursir
part
Ul
y

boil or s

Spinach

Th
It ranks hig
and very nut
flavour to the
Spinach tops
prevent cance
and anti-cancer
beta-carotene ar
vegetable is also
Some of its antio
therefore, be eater
extremely high in o
by person suffering

Sweet Potato

This popular nu
of antioxidant beta-car
Agriculture, about 130 g
about 14 mg of beta-
international units. The lib
heart disease, cataracts, st

Tomato

Tomato is a powerfu
lycopene, a substance that give
in adverse chain reactio
has also been hail
Hopkins

lycopene to be low in those with rectal and bladder cancer. Some consider lycopene a stronger antioxidant than beta-carotene.

Vitamin E-Rich Foods

Vitamin E is high in antioxidant activity. It thus greatly helps protect the heart and arteries. Persons with higher blood levels of vitamin E are less likely to have heart arrhythmia and angina as well as heart attacks. Vitamin E, unlike vitamin C and beta-carotene, is fat-soluble and therefore can help protect fat molecules against disease-causing oxidative damage. Thus for instantce, Vitamin E can effectively counteract oxygen free radical chain reactions that can cut through cells and oxidize their membranes. The presence of vitamin E can stop this damaging chain reaction. "Vitamin E is like a little fire extinguisher in a cell's membrane," says Joe McCord, an antioxidant expert at the University of Colorado. Chief food Sources of Vitamin E are vegetable oils, almonds, soyabeans and sunflower seeds.

Watermelon

The watermelon is one of the most delicious and health-building fruits. The pulp of the fruit is sweet, juicy and soft, with a delicate flavour. It is highly valuable on account of the large amount of easily assimilable sugar contained in its juice. This fruit has high concentration of antioxidants and strong antioxidant activity. It is a major food source of antioxidant and anticancer compounds, lycopene and glutathione. It can thus help prevent damage to cells by oxygen-charged molecules. Watermelon also possesses mild antibacterial and anticoagulant activities.

CHAPTER 8

ANTIVIRAL FOODS

Viruses are particles too small to be seen with a light microscope. They are surrounded by a protein coat. They can reproduce themselves in living cells and cannot exist without ribosomes of the host cell, for they have none themselves. Viruses are responsible for smallpox, poliomyelitis, yellow fever and a number of lesser diseases like cold and influenza. The names given to viruses are in general descriptive, for example herpesviruses and poxviruses. They enter the body through air, water and food, scratches and wounds of the skin.

The foods we eat can determine whether the viruses present in the body are active or passive, starve or flourish, and thus do or do not cause disease. In case of the herpes virus, Richard S. Griffith, M.D., Professor Emeritus of Medicine at Indiana University Medical School, firmly believes that diet determines whether this virus grows, and causes trouble or remains dormant and harmless. It has been shown in lab studies, he says, that the amino acid argentine makes the herpes virus grow, and that the amino acid lysine stops its growth. He opines that lysine wraps itself around the cell, forming a barrier that the virus cannot penetrate.

FOODS THAT FIGHT VIRUSES
Cinnamon, Curd, Dill, Folic Acid Rich Foods, Garlic, Ginger, Grapefruit, Holy Basil, Lemon, Liquid Foods, Long pepper, Onion, Orange and Turmeric.

Cinnamon

The cinnamon is a popular condiment that grows on an evergreen, small and bushy tree in tropical countries. The dried leaves and inner bark are used all over the world as condiment. They have a pleasing fragrant odour and a warm, sweet and aromatic taste.

Cinnamon is an antiviral food and is useful in preventing and treating viral infections. A drink made from it has disinfectant properties. This drink is prepared by putting half a teaspoon of tincture, obtained from the bark of cinnamon tree, in 285 ml of hot water. Taken daily before going into crowded places, it protects against colds and influenza, when these diseases are prevalent in an epidemic form. It also gives a glow of warmth to the whole body.

Cinnamon is also regarded as an effective remedy for sore throat resulting from cold and influenza. One teaspoon of coarsely powdered cinnamon, boiled in a glass of water with a pinch of pepper powder and two teaspoons of honey can be taken as a medicine in the treatment of this condition. Two or three drops of cinnamon oil, mixed with a teaspoon of honey, also give immense relief.

Curd

Curd or yoghurt is a powerful antiviral food. One important reason for this is that it spurs activity of natural killer cells that are particularly vicious in attacking viruses. A daily 225 grams of yoghurt reduced colds and other upper respiratory infections in humans.

The use of curd has also been found beneficial in the treatment of hepatitis and jaundice. Excessive liberation of ammonia, which is one of the major causes of coma in hepatitis, can be prevented by liberal use of curd. The lactic acid organisms in the curd counteract the formation of ammonia. In jaundice, curd or buttermilk sweetened with honey, makes an ideal diet.

Dill

Dill is a green leafy vegetable and a culinary herb. It was known to the ancient Greeks and Romans. Dill leaves are stimulant. They are a soothing medicine and help improve the functioning of the stomach.

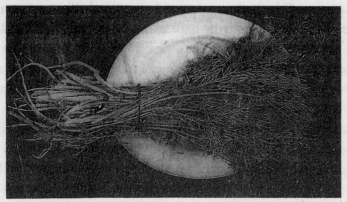

Dill possesses antiviral property and helps fight viruses.

Dill possesses antiviral property and helps fight infection. The seeds of this plant are especially effective in infections like colds and influenza. About 60 grams of infusion of the seeds, mixed with honey, should be given thrice daily in treating these disorders.

Folic Acid Rich Foods

Foods rich in folic acid fight viruses. It is a vitamin of B group and is contained in green leafy vegetables and legumes. In interesting studies of women infected with a virus that can lead to cervical cancer. Charles Butterworth, M.D., at the University of Alabama, discovered that the virus was smashed in the presence of adequate supplies of folic acid.

He further explains that when folic acid is lacking, chromosomes are more likely to break at "fragile" point. This enables the virus to slip into the healthy cells' genetic material, promoting initial changes that precede cancer. Those with low levels of folic acid in their red blood cells were five times more likely to develop such precancerous cell changes than those with higher folic acid levels.

Garlic

Garlic is a potent antiviral food. It works against such viruses as influenza and common cold. It is presumably due to it's ability to produce a warming and drying action generally, leading to stimulation of the blood flow and thereby producing additional energy. Such an increase in overall metabolism may well provide a general strengthening of the overall immune system.

Garlic acts directly against the influenza virus and also stimulates the body's natural defenses against it. In an animal study, researchers fed a garlic extract to mice and then introduced the flu virus into their nasal passages. All the mice that had received the garlic were protected from flu, while the untreated animals all got sick. The researchers presumed that garlic's effect was partly due to its antiviral effect and partly due to its immunity stimulating effect.

Garlic soup is an ancient remedy to reduce the severity of cold. It contains antiseptic and antispasmodic properties, besides several other medicinal virtues. The volatile oil contained in garlic helps to open up the respiratory passages. In soup form, garlic flushes out the system of all toxins and thus helps bring down fever. Garlic oil combined with onion juice, diluted with water and drunk several times a day, has also been found in several studies to be extremely effective in the treatment of common cold.

Some garlic oil products help in curing symptoms of coughs and colds. Garlic has gained this new official credibility mainly through its action in the lungs and sinuses. In the former, it guards against secondary infections, which can arise from the mucosal secretions of a head cold, some of which will end up in lung cavity. While a person's resistance is low from colds or flu, he is likely to get secondary bacterial infection of lung tissue, which means that bronchitis is a potential problem whenever a person gets a really nasty cold. Taking garlic at this time will be very effective as it can often prevent such a possibility.

Garlic is also an effective remedy for herpes virus. Once a person contracted herpes virus, he harbours it for life and it manifests itself when he is in a run down condition. Garlic appears to have an inhibiting effect on cold sores. Even if person has suffered from cold sores for years, this little remedy is well worth a try. Herpes viruses usually infect either oral or genital areas. The usefulness of garlic in combating these serious diseases arises from its antiviral and immunity boosting properties.

Garlic should be used internally as soon as first sign of outbreak of the disease appears. When sores have opened up, the garlic may be applied externally. The most powerful method is to apply garlic juice directly to the sores. Care should however be taken not to irritate the tissues. In the alternative, crushed garlic may be applied in the form of poultice.

Garlic sitz bath may be taken for twenty minutes in case of genital herpes. A garlic clove should be blended or finely chopped and half a litre of boiling water poured over it. It may be allowed to stand for several hours. It should then be poured in the tub filled with enough hot water to cover the hips when the patient sits in it for sitz bath.

Garlic also works against verrucae, which are caused by a virus infection. A thin slice of fresh garlic should be tapped over verrucae with a sticking plaster. It should be changed with a fresh slice each day, and within a week to ten days the verrucae will come away. Certain wart will also respond to this kind of treatment.

A great disadvantage of conventional antibiotics is that they are not effective against viral infections. That is why they do not work against the common cold or flu as well as other serious viral infections. Garlic or its constituents directly kills influenza, herpes and other viruses.

Ginger

Ginger possesses antiviral activity. It destroys influenza viruses. A teaspoon of fresh ginger juice mixed with a cup of fenugreek decoction and honey to taste is an excellent diaphoretic mixture to reduce fever in influenza.

Ginger is also an excellent food remedy for colds and coughs. Ginger should be cut into small pieces and boiled in a cup of water. It should then be strained and half a teaspoon of honey added to it, it should be drunk when hot. Ginger tea, prepared by adding a few pieces of ginger into boiled water before adding the tea leaves, is also an effective remedy for colds and for fevers resulting from cold. It may be taken twice daily.

The use of dry ginger is also considered beneficial in the treatment of mumps. It should be ground to a paste and applied over the swollen parts. As the paste dries, the swelling will reduce and the pain will also subside.

Grapefruit

The juice of this fruit is an antiviral food. Its use has

been found especially valuable in influenza. This juice helps reduce acidity in the system and its bitter properties, arising from a substance called 'maringin', tones up the system and the digestive tract. Grapefruit has also a considerable content of iron, which partly accounts for its distinctly tonic qualities.

Holy Basil

The holy basil is a well-known sacred plant of India. It is a much-branched, erect, stout and aromatic plant. Tradition speaks of this plant from as early as Vedic period. The leaves and seeds of the plant are medicinal.

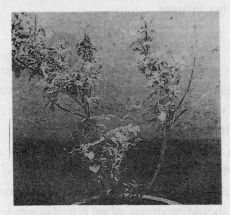

The leaves of Holy Basil are specific for many viral fevers.

The leaves of basil are specific for many viral fevers. During the rainy season, when common cold, influenza and dengue fever are widely prevalent, a decoction of the tender leaves act as a preventive against these diseases. In the case of acute viral fevers, the patients should be given a decoction of the leaves boiled with powdered cardamom in half a litre of water and mixed with honey or jaggery and milk. This brings down the temperature.

For treating influenza, about one gram of the leaves should be boiled along with some ginger in half a litre of water till about half the water is left. This decoction should be taken as tea. The leaves are also beneficial in the treatment of sore throat resulting from cold and influenza. Water boiled with basil leaves should be taken as a drink, and also used as a gargle to get relief from this condition.

Lemon

Lemon possesses antiviral activity. London's first influenza epidemic in November 1931 was cured, not by doctors, but by lemon. Some one has appropriately said, " A lemon a day keeps a cold away." For a bad cold, the juice of two lemons in a half a litre of boiling water, sweetened with honey, taken at bedtime, is a very effective remedy.

Lemon juice is also an excellent remedy in jaundice caused by virus. The patient should be given 20 ml of lemon juice mixed with water, several times a day. This will protect the damaged liver cells.

The juice of lemon is also an effective remedy for measles. It makes an effective thirst-quenching drink in this disease. About 15 to 25 ml of lemon juice should be taken diluted with water for this purpose.

Liquid Foods

In case of cold or influenza, it is always advisable to drink lots of liquids. One good reason for this is that when a person is stuffed up, he breathes through his mouth. As a consequence, the mucous membranes lining the respiratory tract may get dehydrated. Viruses thrive better in these dried environments. Keeping the airway moist through drinking of liquids can discourage them. Hot fluids are better than cold ones as heat can weaken viruses. Dr. Sackner and others have discovered, the vapours from hot water fight congestion to some extent. One should drink at least six to eight glasses of clear liquids a day, including water but not milk, to prevent viruses from becoming active.

Long pepper

Long pepper is good as an antiviral food. Its use has been found very effective in influenza. Half a teaspoon of the powder of long pepper with two teaspoons of honey and half a teaspoon of juice of ginger should be taken thrice a day. It is especially useful in avoiding complications, which follow the onset of the disease, namely, the involvement of the larynx and bronchial tube.

Onion

Onions are an antiviral food. The quercetin, concentrated in it, has antiviral and antibacterial property. This vegetable is thus beneficial in the treatment of several viral diseases, especially cold and influenza. The use of a hot roasted onion before retiring to bed at night is an effective remedy for common cold. For treating influenza, equal amounts of onion juice and honey should be mixed, and three or four teaspoons of this mixture should be taken daily. A French military physician, Dr. Melamet, during the World War II, treated the influenza patients at his hospital at St. Servan by giving them daily from the beginning of their illness the juice of pounded onions three times a day in a warm infusion. Under this treatment the temperature came down within two days and none of the 80 patients so treated died.

Onions are also valuable in warts caused by viral infection. They are irritating to the skin and they stimulate the circulation of the blood. Warts sometimes disappear when rubbed with cut onions.

Orange

This citrus fruit is an antiviral food. As a rich source of antioxidant vitamin C, it has been found beneficial in the treatment of viral diseases like common cold and influenza. Its regular use also helps prevent these diseases. It is most beneficial, when used in the form of juice. The juice is most suitable for all ages and can be taken with advantage in all kinds of viral and other infectious diseases.

The use of orange is also valuable in measles. When the digestive power of the body is seriously hampered, the patient suffers from intense toxaemia, and the lack of saliva coats his tongue and often destroys his thirst for water as well as his desire for food. The agreeable flavour of orange juice helps greatly in overcoming these drawbacks. Orange juice is the most ideal liquid food in this disease.

Turmeric

Turmeric is an antiviral food and helps fight certain viruses. It is especially valuable against influenza virus. A teaspoon of turmeric powder should be mixed in a cup of warm milk and taken three times a day. It prevents complications arising from influenza and also activate the liver, which becomes sluggish during the attack of influenza.

Turmeric is also beneficial in the treatment of measles. Raw roots of turmeric should be dried in the sun and ground to a fine powder. This powder, mixed with a few drops of honey and the juice of few bitter gourd leaves, should be given to the patient suffering from this disease.

CHAPTER 9

BLOOD PRESSURE LOWERING FOODS

High blood pressure is regarded as the silent killer. It is a major maker of heart health. The highest pressure reached during each heartbeat is called systolic pressure and the lowest between two beats is known as diastolic pressure. The blood pressure level considered normal is 120/70, but may go up to 140/90 and still be normal. Within this range, the lower the reading, the better. Blood pressure between 140/90 and 160/95 is considered borderline area. From 160/96 to 180/114, it is classed as moderate hypertension, while 180/115 and upward is considered severe.

Research studies have shown that foods can greatly affect blood pressure. There are certain foods, which may increase blood pressure, while certain others may help lower it. One can thus safely eat once way out of high blood pressure.

FOODS THAT LOWER BLOOD-PRESSURE

Alfalfa, Apple, Bloodwort, Calcium-Rich Foods, Celery, Cucumber, Fruits And Vegetables, Garlic, Indian Goosebery, Olive Oil, Parsley, Potassium-Rich Foods, Potato, Rauwolfia, Rice, Vegetable Juices and Water-Melon Seeds.

Alfalfa

The herbal food, alfalfa helps lower blood pressure. It contains all the elements necessary for the softening of the hardened arteries, which is the main cause for raised blood

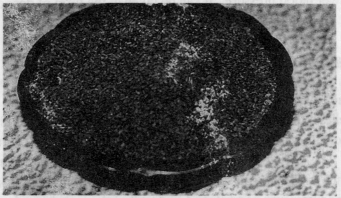

Alfalfa contains all the elements necessary for the softening of the hardened arteries and thus useful in lowering blood pressure.

pressure. Alfalfa can be used in many different forms. The seeds are useful in the form of sprouts. They are delicious and nourishing in salads and soups as well as on sandwiches. Alfalfa can be used in the form of juice extracted from leaves. It is also used extensively in the form of herb tea, which is made from seeds as well as from dried leaves of the plant.

Apple

Apples are considered valuable in lowering blood pressure. They have a rapid and considerable diuretic effect and relive the kidneys by reducing the supply of sodium chloride to a minimum. They also lower the sodium level in the tissues because of the high level of potassium.

Bloodwort

Bloodwort is a bitter, aromatic, stimulant and a tonic herbal food. It induces copious perspiration. The herb is useful in treating high blood pressure. Like all sweat-inducing remedies, bloodwort encourages blood flow to the skin, which helps lower blood pressure.Alkaloid present in bloodwort, is reported to lower blood pressure. It can be taken in the form of decoction or infusion.

Calcium-Rich Foods

Some experts believe that high blood pressure is more due to Calcium deficiency than excess of sodium. They also believe that intake of educate calcium can nullify the blood pressure raising effects of sodium in some patients. According to Dr. David A. Mccarron of Oregon Health Sciences University, some person need more calcium than others to keep blood pressure normal, and quite often those are people who are "salt sensitive," that is, whose blood pressure rises from eating too much sodium.

One theory is that such individuals retain water when they eat too much sodium, and that calcium acts like a natural diuretic to help kidneys release sodium and water, thus reducing blood pressure. Foods rich in Calcium are milk and dairy foods, and green leafy vegetables.

Celery

This vegetable has been used as a folk remedy to lower blood pressure in Asia since ancient times. In a recent study, Dr. William J. Elliot, a pharmacologist at the University of Chicago's Pritzker School of Medicine, isolated a blood-pressure-reducing substance in celery. According to him, celery lowers pressure by reducing blood concentrations of stress hormones that cause blood vessels to constrict. He considered this vegetable to be most effective in those hypertension patients whose blood pressure is linked to mental stress.

Cucumber

The cucumber is one of the oldest known. It is a very popular and widely-cultivated vegetable in is a well-balanced food, which has a cooling and refr. effect. This vegetable contains almost all the essential eleme needed for the preservation of health.

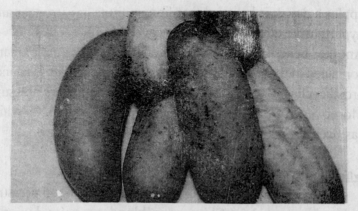

Cucumber is a blood pressure lowering food and its juice is
valuable in high blood pressure.

Cucumber is a blood pressure lowering food. The use of its juice has been found to be an effective food remedy for high blood pressure. A glass of this juice can be taken twice daily, mixed with two teaspoons of honey and a teaspoon of limejuice. This will act as an effective diuretic in treating this disease.

Fruits and Vegetables

A diet rich in fruits and vegetables can lower blood pressure substantially. It has been observed that vegetarians generally suffer less from high blood pressure then non-vegetarians. According to Frank M. Sacks, M.D., an assistant Professor of Medicine at Harvard Medical School, there are certain substances in fruits and vegetables which have

.owers to reduce blood pressure. He considers
. one of such substances, especially in fruits.

.nt Harvard study of nearly 31,000 middle-aged and
.ly persons found that those who ate very little fruit were
.o per cent more likely to develop high blood pressure over
the next four years than men who ate equivalent fibre in five
apples a day. It is believed that fibre in fruits has stronger anti-
hypertensive effect than fibre in vegetables or cereals.

Another benefit of fruits and vegetables is those antioxidants
contained in them increase amounts of hormone-like substance,
prostacyclin, which dilates blood vessels and lowers pressure.
Moreover, fruits and vegetables are rich in vitamin C, which
has been found beneficial in lowering blood pressure.

Garlic

Garlic is an ancient folk remedy to lower blood pressure.
It has been used in China as a blood pressure lowering
medication for a very long time and is now widely used in
Germany for this purpose. It helps reduce blood pressure and
tension because of its power to ease the spasm of the small
arteries. Garlic also slows the pulse, modifies the heart rhythm,
besides relieving the symptoms of dizziness, numbness, shortness
of breath and the formation of gas within the digestive tract.
The average dosage should be two to three capsules a day to
make a dent in the blood pressure.

In a recent German test of Kwai, doses of garlic preparation
equivalent to a couple of garlic cloves daily reduced diastolic
blood pressure in patients with mild high blood pressure. The
blood pressure in the garlic group came down from an average
171/102 to 152/89 after three months, while the blood pressure
of the placebo group remained the same. Interestingly, garlic's
impact increased throughout the test, suggesting that daily

infusions of garlic have a cumulative effect. Both raw and cooked garlic can lower blood pressure, although raw garlic is thought to be more powerful.

Indian Gooseberry

As a super food source of vitamin C, Indian gooseberry is a powerful blood pressure lowering food. A tablespoon each of fresh *amla* juice and honey mixed together should be taken every morning in treating this disease. The use of vitamin C in adequate amount has been found very valuable in lowering blood pressure.

According to researcher Paul F. Jacques, at the U.S. Department of Agriculture's Human Nutrition Research Center on Ageing at Tufts University, a low intake of foods rich in vitamin C predicts high blood pressure.

In one study, he found that elderly people who ate vitamin C equivalent to that in a single orange a day were twice as likely to have high blood pressure as those who ate four times that much. Systolic pressure was eleven points higher and diastolic pressure six points higher among the insufficient vitamin C eaters. In another research, Dr. Jacques concluded that low blood levels of vitamin C raised systolic pressure about 16 per cent and diastolic pressure 9 per cent.

"There is something about not eating enough vitamin C that raises blood pressure" says Dr. Jacques. Thus, if a person has high blood pressure, he should eat vitamin C at least the amount contained in an orange a day. Dr. Jacques also believes that other components in fruits and vegetables, besides vitamin C, also help keep blood pressure in check. Foods rich in vitamin C, besides Indian Gooseberry, are Citrus fruit, green leafy vegetables, sprouted Bengal and green grams.

Olive Oil

The use of olive oil has been found beneficial in the treatment of high blood pressure. A study, by researchers at Stanford medical school, of 76 middle-aged men with high blood pressure a few years ago, concluded that the amount of monounsaturated fat in three tablespoons of olive oil a day could lower systolic pressure about nine points and diastolic pressure by six points. More remarkable, a University of Kentucky study found that a mere two-thirds of a tablespoon of olive oil daily reduced blood pressure by about five systolic points and four diastolic points in men.

Parsley

Parsley is one of the oldest and best-known vegetables. It was known to ancient Romans. It is high in vitamin and mineral contents. This vegetable is especially rich in ascorbic acid and hence is a good blood cleanser. Raw parsley juice has properties, which are essential to oxygen metabolism in maintaining the normal action of the adrenal and thyroid glands. Parsley is a blood pressure lowering food. It contains elements which help maintain the blood vessels, particularly the capillaries and arterial system in a healthy condition. It may be taken as a beverage by simmering it gently in the water for a few minutes and drinking it several times daily. Alternatively, it may be taken in the form of juice extracted from the leaves.

Potassium-Rich Foods

Foods rich in potassium have been found beneficial in lowering blood pressure. Potassium is a strong medicine for high blood pressure. Adding potassium to the diet can lower blood pressure and reducing potassium can raise it. Thus, eating a low-potassium diet can cause high blood pressure.

This was proved, in a test at Temple University School of Medicine. In this test, 10 men with normal blood pressure ate a potassium-adequate diet and then a potassium-restricted diet, each for nine days. Deprived of potassium, the men experienced an average raise in arterial pressure, including both diastolic and systolic pressure, of 4.1 points – up from 90.9 to 95. Their blood pressure shot even higher when the men's diets were full of sodium. Thus, potassium also helps keep a high-sodium diet in check, said the study's senior author, G. Gopal Krishna, M.D. He believed that too little potassium leads to sodium retention, which over a period may trigger high blood pressure. Taking enough potassium can also reduce the doses of medication a person needs. A study at the University of Naples in Italy discovered that after a year on high-potassium diet, 81 per cent of a group of patients needed only half their original dosages of drugs to control their high blood pressure. Further, 38 per cent of the high-potassium group was able to stop medication entirely. They simply ate three to six servings of high-potassium foods a day, boosting their average intake of potassium about 60 per cent.

Potassium is widely distributed in foods. All vegetables, especially green leafy vegetables, grapes, orange, lemon, raisins, whole grains, lentils, sunflower seeds, nuts, milk, cottage cheese and butter milk are rich sources.

Potato

The potato, especially in boiled form, is a valuable food for lowering blood pressure. When boiled with their skins, potatoes absorb very little salt. Thus they can form a useful addition to a salt free diet recommended for patients with high blood pressure. They are rich in potassium but not in sodium salts. The magnesium present in this vegetable exercises beneficial effect in lowering blood pressure.

Rauwolfia

Rauwolfia is an erect plant with a smooth stem. The drug consists of the dried roots with their bark intact, preferably collected in autumn from three or four year old plants.

Rauwolfia is one of the best remedies for high blood pressure, and it has been adopted by medical fraternity in most countries, especially America. The alkaloids contained in this herb, which have a direct effect on hypertension, have been isolated from it and are widely used by the practitioners of modern medicine. But they have certain unpleasant side effects, which the drug taken in its raw form, does not have. Practitioners of the Ayurvedic medicine preferred to use its root in a powdered form. Half a teaspoon of this powder, taken thrice a day, is effective in relieving hyper-tension.

Renowned Ayurvedic physicians of Calcutta, Dr. Gannath Sen and Dr. Kartik Chandra Bose made experiments with rauwolfia in cases of high blood pressure and extreme type of insanity attended by grave signs of absurdity of the mind. The powder of its root in 12 to 20 decigrams dose not only provided a sedative effect but lowered the blood pressure as well. Patients in most cases regain normal senses within a week but some, however, require longer treatment. These physicians found the result most encouraging in cases of high blood pressure where it does not produce any untoward changes like thickening of the walls of the nerves.

Rice

Rice has a low-fat, low-cholesterol and low-salt content. It makes a perfect diet for those hypertensive persons who have been advised salt-restricted diet. Calcium in brown rice, in particular, soothes and relaxes the nervous system and helps relieve the symptoms of high blood pressure.

Vegetable Juices

Raw vegetable juices, especially carrot and spinach juices, constitute a powerful blood pressure lowering food. They can be taken separately or in combination in treating high blood pressure. If taken in combination, 300ml of carrot juice and 200ml of spinach juice should be mixed together.

Watermelon Seeds

The seeds of watermelon can help lower blood pressure. They are a valuable safeguard against high blood pressure. According to Dr. Foster, an eminent physician, the nation-wide use of watermelon seeds by the Chinese may be an important factor in the low blood pressure among them. The Chinese dry and roast the seeds and consume them liberally. In a recent experiment, a substance extracted from watermelon seeds was shown to have a definite action in dilating the blood vessels and this helps lower blood pressure.

In India, watermelon seeds are being used in medicine from ancient times as a base in many Unani and Ayurvedic tonic preparations. Seeds contain a glucoside known as cucurbotrine. Milky juice of the seeds obtained by grinding them and straining through a cloth is used in high blood pressure and many other diseases with beneficial results. Adding few almonds and a teaspoon of poppy seeds to a tablespoon of watermelon seeds, and ground to get the milk, is more effective in treating high blood pressure. Honey may be added to taste. Regular use of this milk from the seeds protects the arterial lumen.

CHAPTER 10

CALMING AND SEDATIVE FOODS

There are certain natural foods, which may work as sedatives by stimulating the activity and levels of neurotransmitters, such as serotonin that calms the brain. Honey and other carbohydrates are considered by some to affect serotonin, inducing tranquillity and sleep in most people. Glucose may also work directly on the neurons in the brain's hypothalamus. There are certain other foods that contain peptides or release peptides in the gut that can send messages from the intestinal tract directly to the nervous system and brain.

FOODS THAT INDUCE TRANQUILLITY AND SLEEP

Aniseed, Bottle gourd, Celery, Cumin seeds, Dill, Honey, Indian Hemp, Lettuce, Long pepper, Milk, Nutmeg, Oats, Poppy Seeds, Rauwolfia Thiamin-Rich Foods and Valerian.

Aniseed

Aniseed is an annual culinary herb belonging to *ajwain* or celery family. Its fruit, known as aniseed, is one of the oldest spices. The seed is ground-gray to grayish–brown in colour, oval in shape and 3.2 to 4.8 mm in length. It has an agreeable odour and a pleasant taste.

Aniseed is a calming and sedative food. A tea made from this spice can calm the nerves and induce sleep. This tea is prepared by boiling about 375 ml of water in a vessel and adding a teaspoon of aniseed. The water should be covered with a lid and drunk hot or warm. The tea may be sweetened with honey and hot milk may also be added to it. This tea should be taken after meals or before going to bed. Aniseed should not be boiled too long as it may lose its digestive properties and essential oils during the process.

Bottle Gourd

The bottle gourd, also known as wild gourd, is a common vegetable in India. It is yellowish-green, having the shape of a bottle. It has white pulp, with white seeds embedded in its spongy flesh.

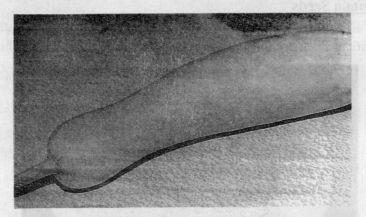

Bottle Gourd is a relaxing and sedative food and it imparts tranquility after eating it.

This vegetable is relaxing and sedative food. It imparts tranquillity and a feeling of relaxation after eating it. It is thus an effective remedy for sleeplessness. A mixture of bottle gourd and sesame oil can also be beneficially massaged over the scalp every night before retiring, to induce sleep. The cooked leaves of bottle gourd, taken as a vegetable, also serve as sedative and calming food. They are thus valuable in insomnia. The bottle gourd should not be eaten in raw form as it may prove harmful for stomach and intestine.

Celery

This vegetable is of great value as a calming and sedative food. It can be beneficially used in sleeplessness. The juice of Celery leaves, mixed with a tablespoon of honey, should be taken at night before retiring. It will help one to relax into a soothing and restful sleep. Celery seeds also exercise calming and soothing effect. The essential oil contained in them has a specific effect on the regulation of the nervous system and has a great calming influence.

Cumin Seeds

Cumin Seeds exercise soothing effect on the nervous system. They are thus valuable in insomnia. A teaspoon of the

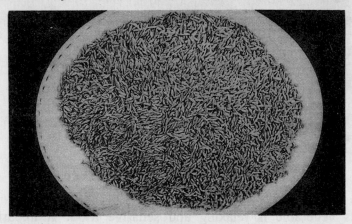

Cumin seeds exercise soothing effects in the nervous system and are thus valuable in insomnia.

fried powder of cumin seeds and the pulp of the ripe banana,

ies and Africa since time imm
yne properties of Indian hemp w
edical men in the early years of the
orporated in the British and United
is used as a drug to reduce excitement,
l as to induce deep sleep. The leaves
nistered to induce sleep where opium
, which is an active ingredient of hemp,
e drugs to induce deep sleep.

t is a highly calming and sedative food. It
ing sleep. It contains a sleep inducing
ctucarium'. The juice of this plant has been
the sedative action of opium without the
itement. Liberal intake of this juice is thus
insomnia. The seeds of lettuce in the form of
o useful in this disease.

ular herb is a calming and sedative food. Its use
l highly beneficial in the treatment of nervous
ers like insomnia, epilepsy, convulsions and
ould be taken in doses of three to five decigrams
with honey.

is one of the most commo
t the world. It occupies a uniq
ce of health and healing diseases.
rded as a complete food as it co
rates, all the known vitamins, variou

Honey

Honey is a ~~valuable~~ sedative food. It ha~~s~~ tranquillising propertie~~s~~ has hypnotic action in ~~the~~ with water, before going ~~to bed in~~ a big cup of water. Bab~~ies~~ honey. It should, however, ~~not be given before one~~ year of age, as there is a dan~~ger~~

~~Indi~~an Hemp

The leaves of the hemp pl~~ant~~ ~~f~~ood. Preparations of In~~dian~~

Long Pepper

This popu~~lar spice~~ has been foun~~d~~ system disor~~ders~~ hysteria. It sh~~ould~~ daily, mixed ~~with~~

Milk

Milk ~~is used~~ throughou~~t~~ maintenan~~ce~~ It is rega~~rded~~ carbohyd~~rates~~

the food ingredients considered essential for sustaining life and maintaining health.

Milk possesses calming and sedative properties. It is a rich source of amino acid tryptophan. This amino acid relaxes the nervous system and induces sleep. Milk is thus, very valuable in insomnia. A glass of milk, sweetened with honey, should be taken every night before going to bed in treating this condition. It acts as a tonic and a tranquilliser. Massaging the milk over the soles of the feet has also been found effective in treating this condition.

Nutmeg

This popular spice possesses sedative and calming properties. It is an effective medicine for sleeplessness. The powder of nutmeg, mixed with fresh *amla* juice, should be taken in treating this condition. This mixture also forms an effective remedy for mental irritability and depression. Nutmeg powder can also be taken mixed with milk.

Nutmeg paste, mixed with honey, can be given with beneficial results as a sedative medicine to those infants who keep on crying the whole night without any obvious reason. It should, however, not be given regularly without medical advice as it may cause serious complications and addiction.

Oats

This popular cereal induces tranquillity and sleep. It possesses calming and sedative properties. These properties emanate from oatmeal. A tea made from oats is especially valuable in cases of chronic headaches. It also makes a good bedtime drink for those who are unable to sleep as well as for those who are suffering from nervous exhaustion. Excessive use of oats should, however, be avoided as high doses may cause gas, abdominal bloating and pain.

Poppy Seeds

Poppy seeds are found in poppy heads. They form part of many prescriptions for tonics. The plant is endowed with roots of strong fragrance. Poppy seeds are of great value as a calming and sedative food. The seeds can be beneficially used as a valuable medicine in sleeplessness. About 30 grams of milk extracted from the seeds mixed with honey can be used for treating this condition. A teaspoon of poppy seed oil taken every night is also very effective in sleeplessness.

Rauwolfia

This popular Indian medicinal plant is a calming and sedative food. It is thus effective in treating insomnia. The hypnotic action of the drug appears to have been known since ancient times. The very first dose of rauwolfia enables the patient of a phlegmatic and gouty nature to go to sleep.

The powder of the root in a quantity of 0.25 grams to 0.50 grams should be mixed with some scented substance like cardamom and given to the patient at bedtime. The patient will have a sound sleep during the entire night. In case of chronic insomnia, the patient should take 0.25 grams twice a day, both in the morning and at night before retiring.

Thiamin-Rich Foods

Of the various food elements, thaimine or vitamin B_1 is of special significance as a calming and sedative substance. Its use has, therefore, been found very valuable in inducing sleep. This vitamin is vital for strong and healthy nerves. A body starved of thaimine over a long period will be unable to relax and fall asleep naturally. Rich sources of this vitamin are whole grain cereals, pulses and nuts.

Valerian

Valerian is an ancient popular medicinal plant, with strong calming and sedative properties. It is a traditional remedy for functional disturbances of the nervous system. It was perhaps the earliest treatment of neurosis, accompanied by physical diseases with mental symptoms or social maladjustment, especially in interpersonal relationships.

The herb is particularly useful in treating cases of hysteria, restless and irritable conditions. The drug exercises depressant action on the overall central nervous system. It has gained importance in recent years owing to its beneficial effects in epilepsy.

The herb is useful in inducing sleep due to its sedative property. It reduces excitement, irritation and pain. The fresh juice of the plant can be used beneficially as a narcotic in insomnia.

The juice of the fresh rhizomes and roots is considered more effective in the treatment of nervous disorders as its medicinal properties get reduced on drying. An infusion of valerian is prepared by infusing 80 grams of the herb in half a litre of boiling water. The later should be taken in small quantities, three or four times daily.

CHAPTER 11

CANCER FIGHTING FOODS

Diet is now considered a major factor in prevention and treatment of cancer. According to the American National Cancer Institute, about one-third of all types of cancers are linked to diet. Thus, right choice of foods can help prevent a majority of new cancer cases and deaths from cancer. Cancer usually develops over a long period. Latest researches show that what one eats may interfere with cancer development process at various stages, from conception to growth and spread of the cancer. Foods can block the chemical activation, which normally initiates cancer. Antioxidants, including vitamins, can eradicate carcinogens and can even repair some of the cellular damage caused by them. Cancers that are in the process of growth can also be prevented from further spreading by judicial selection of foods. Even in advanced cases, the right foods can prolong the patient's life.

FOODS THAT CONTROL AND PREVENT CANCER

Beet Juice, Cabbage And Other Cruciferous Vegetables, Carrot, Citrus Fruits, Curd, Fiber-Rich Foods, Fruits And Vegetables, Garlic And Onion, Grapes, Green Vegetables, Indian Gooseberry, Liquorice, Margosa, Milk, Olive Oil, Papaya Leaves, Raw Foods, Soyabeans, Tomato, Vitamin C and A-Rich Foods, Wheat Bran and Wheat Grass Juice.

... of
... bolism
... that less
... revealed by
... chnovicz and
... search **in New**

... indoles in these
... process in which the
... type of oestrogen that
... ists on women and men, the
... p" the oestrogen-deactivation
... , says Dr. Michnovicz. The test
... people would ordinarily eat:
... , butinol, the amount in about
... age, ... less would also burn up
... lesser degree. ... own that women with
... gen metabolism ha... yer risks of hormone-
... ancers, such as breast, u... ne and endometrial
... s Dr. Michnovicz.
... of cabbage in its raw form has also been found
... ole in preventing colon cancer, according to Dr. ...
... ke at the U.S. Department of Agriculture, who has a colon
... mily history of colon cancer. Dr. Duke says his ... ge every
... polps decreased dramatically after he ate raw cabbage
... oter day.

...rrot This vegetable, as a super food source of beta-
... rotene, has been found valuable in preventing lung cancer.
... eta-carotene is an orange pigment isolated from ca...
... ore than 150 years ago. It acts as an antid...

type of cancer. These vegetables
oestrogen from the body. It also
of oestrogen, that is, burning
of it is available to feed ca
the research studies cond
colleagues at the Insti
York City.
These studies in
cruciferous veg
body deactiva
cabb romot
process
dose

be advisable to extra

markedly in

Cabbage and Other Cruciferous Vege

Cabbage and other cruciferous vege
cauliflower and brussels sprouts are som
important foods, which may help immunize
cancer by managing oestrogen, a known prom

Beet Juice

The juice of red beet possesses anticancer property and is thus considered beneficial in the prevention and treatment of cancer. It is one of the best vegetable juices and a rich source of natural sugar. It contains sodium, potassium, phosphorus, calcium, sulphur, chlorine, iodine, iron, copper, vitamin B_1, B_2, niacin, B_6, C and P. This juice stimulates the liver and its detoxifying activity is of great value in treating cancer.

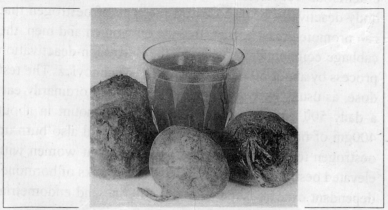

The juice of red beet possesses anticancer property and is thus useful in the prevention and treatment of cancer.

Half a glass of this juice can be taken three times daily. Lactic acid fermented and a well balance beet juice will markedly increase the oxygenation of the body cells. It would be advisable to extract juice both from roots and tops.

Cabbage and Other Cruciferous Vegetables

Cabbage and other cruciferous vegetables like broccoli, cauliflower and brussels sprouts are some of the most important foods, which may help immunize against breast cancer by managing oestrogen, a known promoter of this type of cancer. These vegetables hasten the removal of oestrogen from the body. It also speeds up the metabolism of oestrogen, that is, burning up the hormone so that less of it is available to feed cancer. This has been revealed by the research studies conducted by Dr. Jon Michnovicz and colleagues at the Institute of Hormone Research in New York City.

These studies indicate that specific indoles in these cruciferous vegetables accelerate a process in which the body deactivates or disposes off the type of oestrogen that can promote breast cancer. In tests on women and men, the cabbage compound "turned up" the oestrogen-deactivation process by about 50 per cent, says Dr. Michnovicz. The test dose, as usual, exceeded what people would ordinarily eat: a daily 500 mg of indole-3-carbinol, the amount in about 400gm of raw cabbage, but eating less would also burn up oestrogen to a lesser degree. It is known that women with elevated oestrogen metabolism have lower risks of hormone-dependant cancers, such as breast, uterine and endometrial cancer says Dr. Michnovicz.

The use of cabbage in its raw form has also been found valuable in preventing colon cancer, according to Dr. Jim Duke at the U.S. Department of Agriculture, who has a family history of colon cancer. Dr. Duke says his colon polyps decreased dramatically after he ate raw cabbage every other day.

Carrot

This vegetable, as a super food source of beta-carotene, has been found valuable in preventing lung cancer. Beta-carotene is an orange pigment isolated from ca~ more than 150 years ago. It acts as an antid~

cancer. A recent study at the State University of New York at Buffalo shows that eating beta-carotene-rich vegetables more than once a week dramatically decreased lung cancer odds when compared with non-eaters of this vegetable. Munching a single raw carrot at least twice a week reduces lung cancer by 60 per cent. The anti cancer power of beta-carotene comes from both its antioxidant capabilities and its ability to enhance immunological defenses, which is important in preventing and controlling cancer.

The juice extracted from carrot is considered a miracle juice. It has been found highly beneficial in the prevention and treatment of cancer. Mary C. Hogle, a graduate of the University of Kansas and an experienced student of nutrition and food chemistry, claims to have been cured by a carrot juice regime, in combination with bland foods, when it had been thought that she was incurable. In her book, Food that Alkalize and Heal, she gives a short history of her case and some very fine suggestions on what to eat and how to prepare certain broths and bland foods. She firmly believes that carrot juice is one of the most potent alkalizers. She says, "The excellence of carrot juice as a source of vitamin A no doubt explains much of its health value. Vitamin A has been called the anti-infective vitamin and it has as its specific function the resisting and correcting of all infection of the epithelial surfaces, which include the skin covering, the mucous membranes and all the glands. Vitamin A is considered one of the main elements, in a basic way, to protect all infections."

She further says about carrot, "Carrot juice has established itself as the peer of all as a rapid alkalizer. This is no doubt partly because the contained alkalies are easily appropriated by the body and partly because juice can generally be consumed in large quantities without unpleasant or harmful effects."

Citrus Fruits

Citrus fruits like grapefruit, lime, lemon and orange possess powerful anti-cancer properties. According to toxicologist Herbert Pierson, Ph.D., a diet and cancer expert formally with the American National Cancer Institute, regards citrus fruits as a total anti-cancer package, because they possess every class of natural substances like carotenoids, flavonoids, terpenes, limonoids and coumarins, which have individually helped neutralize powerful chemical carcinogens in animals.

One analysis found that citrus fruits possess 58 known anti-cancer chemicals, more than any other food. Further, Dr. Pierson says, "The beauty of citrus is that several classes of phytochemicals are highly likely to act more powerfully...as a natural mixture than when they appear separately." In other words, whole citrus fruits are a marvelous combination of anti-cancer compounds. One such anti-cancer compound is glutathione. Whole oranges contain high concentrations of this tested disease-fighting compound. However, when extracted, the juice tends to lose glutathione concentrations. Oranges also are the highest of all foods by far in glucarate, another cancer-inhibitor. Some experts ascribe the dramatic decline of stomach cancer in the United States to the wider use of citrus fruits.

Curd

Curd or yoghurt is a powerful preventive against colon cancer. It is a rich source of vitamin D and calcium, these two nutrients are highly valuable in preventing cancer.

Research studies show that lactobacillus acidophilus helps suppress enzyme activity needed to convert otherwise harmless substances into cancer-causing chemicals in the colon. This has been proved by studies done by leading researchers Barry R.Goldin and Sherwood L Gorbach at the New England Medical Centre. For a month, volunteers drank two glasses of plain milk everyday. Then they took acidophilus milk. Researchers measured the enzyme activity in the subjects' colon. Drinking acidophilus milk caused dangerous enzyme activity to drop by 40-80 per cent. This means certain carcinogenic activity in the colon was remarkably suppressed.

Fiber-Rich Foods

Fiber-rich foods help fight Cancer. According to an expert, Dr. Greenwald, fibre-rich vegetables can reduce the risk of colon cancer. His analysis of 37 studies done in the last 20 years showed that eating high-fibre foods or vegetables cut the chances of colon cancer by 40 per cent. The most significant food sources of fibre are unprocessed wheat bran, whole cereals such as wheat, rice, barley; legumes such as potato, carrots, beat, turnip and sweet potato; fruits like mango and guava and leafy vegetables such as cabbage, lettuce and celery.

Fruits and Vegetables

Researches conducted in ascertaining links between diet and cancer since 1970 have now conclusively proved that fruits and vegetables can serve as antidote to cancer. The normal servings of fruits and vegetables are two fruits and three vegetables a day. Adding more fruits and vegetables to these servings can reduce the risk of cancer. One serving means 100-115gm of cooked or chopped raw fruit or vegetables, 70-85gm of raw leafy vegetables, one medium piece of fruit, or 170ml of fruit juice or vegetable juice.

Garlic and Onions

More than 30 different compounds have been isolated from garlic and onions, which are potent enemies of carcinogens. These compounds include diallyl sulphide, quercetin and ajoene. In animals, they block the most terrifying cancer-causing agents such as nitrosamines and aflatoxin, linked specifically to stomach, lung and liver cancer. Feeding garlic to animals consistently blocks cancer. Harvard scientists immunized hamsters against certain cancers by putting ground onions in their drinking water.

One of the leading researcher on garlic, Michael Wargovich, at Houston's M. D., Anderson Cancer Center, gave some mice purified diallyl sulphide from garlic and others plain mice food, followed by powerful carcinogens. Mice eating the garlic substance had 75 per cent fewer colon tumours. More impressive, when given agents that cause oesophageal cancer in mice, not a single one getting the diallyl sulphide got with cancer. Similarly, John Milner, Head of Nutrition at Penn State University, blocked 70 per cent of breast tumours in mice by feeding them fresh garlic. In humans, studies show that those who eat more onions and garlic are less prone to various cancers.

Garlic may also interfere with the progress of the cancer. A recent German study found that garlic compounds are toxic to malignant cells. Thus, garlic substances might help destroy cancerous cells somewhat the way chemotherapy drugs do. In the German study of human cells, one potent garlic compound, ajoene, was three times as toxic to malignant cells as to normal cells.

Garlic might also discourage colon and stomach cancers by functioning as an antibiotic. New research studies suggest that an infection by H.pylori bacteria contributes to these cancers. If so, says Dr. Tim Byers of the Centers for Disease Control and Prevention; garlic might fight cancer by attacking the bacteria.

Grapes

About 125 years ago, Dr. Lambe, a pioneer reformer and dietitian, treated cancer with grapes in England. In recent times, Johanna Brandt, discovered for herself that cancer could be treated successfully with exclusive grape diet. This discovery was made by her, while experimenting on herself by fasting and dieting alternately, in the course of her nine-year battle against cancer. She claimed to have cured herself by this mode of treatment. The effectiveness of exclusive grape diet in treating cancer is attributable to the presence of generous quantities of salts of potash in grapes. It has been noted that there is a marked deficiency of potash in the average cancer patient.

In the treatment of cancer by exclusive diet of grapes, the patient should drink plenty of pure cooled water for first three days. He should undertake lukewarm water enema daily with the strained juice of lemon during this period. After the short fast, the patient should have a grape meal every two hours from 8 a.m. to 8 p.m. This should be followed for a week or two, even a month or two, in chronic cases of long standing. The patient should begin the grape cure with a small quantity. He should increase the quantity of grapes gradually so as to take 200 grams at a meal in course of time.

Green vegetables

Green vegetables, especially green leafy vegetables, exhibit extraordinarily broad anti-cancer powers. A recent Italian study showed a remarkable protection from the frequent consumption of green vegetables against the risk of most cancers. The green vegetables, such as spinach, dark green lettuce and broccoli, are full of many different antioxidants, including beta-carotene and folic acid. These vegetables also contain lutein, a little-known antioxidant, which is considered as powerful as beta-carotene in preventing cancer.

To get green vegetables with most carotenoids, and other anti-cancer agents, the darkest green vegetables should be selected. According to Frederick Khachik, Ph.D., a research scientist at the Department of Agriculture, 'The darker green they are the most cancer-inhibiting carotenoids they have." He also says lutein and other carotenoids are not lost during cooking or freezing, although heat does harm more fragile antioxidants, including vitamin C and glutathione.

Indian Gooseberry

Indian goosebery, as a super food source of vitamin C, can be beneficially used in the fight against cancer. Vitamin C is the most potent anti-toxin known. It can effectively neutrilise or minimize the damaging effect of most chemical carcinogens in food and environment and, thus, be of great value in cancer prevention programs, as well as in the treatment of cancer. Repeated laboratory tests at Coonoor shows that every 100 grams of fresh indian goosebery provides 470 to 680 mg of vitamin C.

The dehydrated berry is especially beneficial in controlling cancer, as vitamin C value of *amla* increases greatly when the juice is extracted from the fruit. The dehydrated berry provides 2428 to 3470 mg of vitamin C per 100 grams.

Even when it is dried in shade and turned into powder, it retains as much as 1780 to 2660 mg of vitamin C.

Liquorice

Liquorice, a popular spice and a flavouring agent, is an anti-cancer food. It has the properties, which not only help prevent cancer but also retard its spread. Triterpenoids

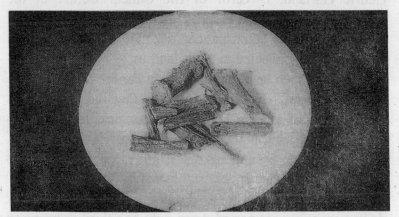

Liquorice has the property which, not only helps prevent cancer but also retard its spread.

contained in liquorice may block quick-growing cancer cells and cause some pre-cancerous cells to return to normal growth. This spice can be used either in the form of powder, decoction or infusion. These preparations can be taken mixed with honey.

Margosa

The use of margosa leaves is considered beneficial as a supportive treatment of cancer according to Ayurveda. From the point of view of this system of medicine, the blood gets toxicated and body heat increases in this disease. Margosa leaves help in purifying the blood and in reducing body heat. The patient should therefore chew 10-12 margosa leaves daily in the morning.

Milk

Milk as a rich source of vitamin D and calcium, is an important food, which can reduce the risk of colon cancer. Both these nutrients are potential cancer suppressor. Dr. Cedric Garland, Director of the Cancer Centre at the University of California at San Diego, says vitamin D blood levels can predict colon cancer risk. He examined 25,620 blood samples collected in Maryland in 1974 for vitamin D content, and then he compared colon cancer rates over the next eight years. His conclusion was that those with high blood levels of vitamin D were 70 per cent less likely to develop colon cancer then those with low levels.

Calcium appears to suppress disastrous physiological events leading to colon cancer, as established by some studies. Dr. Garland has noted that men who drank two glasses of milk daily over a 20-year period were only one-third as prone to developing colon cancer as non-milk drinkers. Dr. Garland estimates that 1,200-1,400 mg of calcium per day might prevent as much as 65-75 per cent of colon cancers. One reason is that calcium can suppress the proliferation of surface cells on the inner lining of the colon, thereby preventing the rapid cell growth that is a sign of developing cancer.

Rich sources of calcium, besides milk and milk products are, whole wheat, leafy vegetables such as lettuce, spinach, and cabbage, carrot, watercress, orange, lemon, almond, fig and walnut.

Olive Oil

The use of olive oil is considered beneficial in the

prevention and treatment of cancer. Eating too much fat has been linked with breast cancer. This has been adequately proved by a research study on 750 Italian women. It was found in this study that the women who eat the most saturated fats had three times the risk of breast cancer compared with those eating the least. Eating too much fat can influence the spread and harshness of an existing breast cancer, its recurrence and survival chances. Some researches show that the more the saturated animal fat in the diet, the greater the odds of axillary lymph node involvement or spread of the cancer, and the more the total fat in a diet, the greater the chances of dying from breast cancer. Mediterranean women who eat lots of olive oil have low rates of breast cancer, as do Japanese women who eat lots of fish oils but little animal fat. In countries where animal fat consumption is high, breast cancer rates are also high.

Papaya Leaves

Success in the treatment of cancer has been claimed by a 74-year old lady from Australia by the use of leaves of papaya, a delicious tropical fruit, in a letter to "Weekend Bulletin", Gold coast, Australia. She had undergone a surgical operation for her bladder cancer, but cancer could not be completely removed. While undergoing further treatment in Brisbane, she used papaya leaves and subsequently used boiled skin of papaya, when her stock of leaves had run out. After 3 months, when she went to her doctor for a checkup, it was found that her cancer had been healed. In U.S.A. also, the American scientist Dr. Jerry McLaughlin of the University of Purdue, used papaya in the fight against cancer. According to him, he has found a chemical component in the papaya tree that is "one million times stronger than the strongest anti-cancer medicine." There are many reports that cancer sufferers have been healed by drinking papaya leaf concentrate.

Raw Foods

Dr. Kirstine Nolfi of Denmark, who herself suffered from cancer, found by experiment the value of raw foods in treating cancer. She recovered from this dreaded disease after treating herself with an exclusive diet of raw foods and then opened an institution called Humlegarden. She attained great success in treating cancer patients at this institution and wrote a book about her success. In her book Dr. Nolfi tells how, whenever she slipped off her raw food diet or used salt, the condition reappeared with renewed vigor. Then when she went back to the raw food diet and stuck to it, the cancer subsided. This experience shows that cancer cannot be cured but it can be prevented and held under control by a raw juice and raw food diet. Dr. Nolfi gave a great deal of credit to raw garlic and raw potatoes, which she claims were the key vegetables in the success of the raw food diet.

Soyabeans

This vegetable contains compounds, which can manipulate oestrogen and also directly inhibit the growth of cancerous cells, thereby reducing the risk of breast cancer in women of all ages, according to Stephen Barnes, Ph.D., associate professor of pharmacology and biochemistry at the University of Alabama. One soyabean compound, phyto-estrogens is quite similar chemically to the drug tamoxifen, given to certain women to help prevent breast cancer and its spread. Soyabean also helps block the growth of cancer cells in another way, not related to oestrogen. Studies in cells have found that soyabean compounds, for mysterious reasons, can entirely halt the growth of cancerous cells even though they do not have any oestrogen receptors to block, according to Dr. Barnes. That means these soyabean compounds fight cancer in at least two separate ways, he says.

Soyabeans can be used in various forms such as milk, curd, flours, green beans, sprouts and oil. The soyabean milk is the main article of food and it can be converted into several other food products like curd, casein, sweets and pudding. The soya flour is the most widely used product of soyabean. It is prepared by first roasting the soyabean and removing their coatings. They are then turned into powder.

Tomato

Tomato is regarded as an anti-cancer food. Its lycopene, which gives this vegetable its color, is the main ingredient. This ingredient helps prevent cancer. A research study conducted by Dr. Helmut Sies of Germany has found that lycopene is twice as powerful as beta-carotene at "quenching singlet oxygen," an unchecked toxic oxygen molecule that can trigger cancer in cells. Tomatoes are the major source of lycopene in the food supply, and that includes all types of tomato products, such as cooked tomatoes, canned tomatoes and sauces, tomato paste and ketchup. Lycopene is also highly concentrated in watermelon.

Vitamin C and A-Rich Foods

Recent research has shown that certain vitamins can be successfully employed in the fight against cancer and that they can increase the life expectancy of some terminal cancer patients. According to recent Swedish studies, vitamin C in large doses can be effective prophylactic agent against cancer. Noted Japanese scientist, Dr. Fukunir Mirishige and his colleagues have recently found that a mixture of vitamin C and copper compound has lethal effects on cancer.

Foods rich in vitamin C are Indian Gooseberry, citrus fruits, green leafy vegetables and sprouted Bengal and green grams.

According to several studies, vitamin A exerts an inhibiting effect on carcinogenesis. It is one of the most important aids to the body's defense system to fight and prevent cancer. Dr. Leonida Santamaria and his colleagues at the University of Pavis in Italy have uncovered preliminary evidence suggesting that beta-carotene, a precursor of vitamin A, may actually inhibit skin cancer by helping the body nullify the cancer-causing process known as oxidation.

Foods rich in vitamin A are whole milk, curds, butter, pumpkin, carrots, green leafy vegetables, tomatoes, papaya and mango.

Wheat Bran

One way to reduce the chances of breast cancer is to curtail oestrogen levels in the blood. It can be achieved by taking wheat bran cereals. Wheat bran has specific property to lower dramatically the circulating levels of cancer-promoting oestrogen in the blood. This was found in a research study by David P. Rose, M.D., of the American Health Foundation in New York. Some women were made to eat three to four high-fibre muffins a day made with oat bran, corn bran or wheat bran. That doubled their fibre intake from about 15g to 30g. After a month, there was a little difference in their blood oestrogen levels, but after two months, oestrogen levels had come down by about 17 per cent in the women eating wheat bran. Oestrogen levels did not change in eaters of oat bran or corn bran muffins. However all type of brans, including wheat bran as rich sources of fibre can help reduce the risk of colon cancer. Some specific foods, however, have shown outstanding powers in this regard. Wheat bran has the best reputation as a formidable colon cancer fighter.

Wheat Grass Juice

Dr. Ann Wigmore of Boston, U.S.A., the well-known naturopath and pioneer in the field of living food nutrition, has been testing the effect of a drink made of fresh wheatgrass in the treatment of leukaemia. She claims to have cured several cases of this disease by this method. Dr. Wigmore points out that by furnishing the body with live minerals, vitamins, trace elements and chlorophyll, the wheatgrass juice may help repair the damaged cells.

In adopting this mode of treatment, the patient should undertake fast on wheat grass for seven days. This fast provides the body with all the nutrients of the richest living food in a form so concentrated and easy to digest that it provides virtually all the benefits of a complete fast with none of the dangers of total abstinence. Such a fast can be pleasantly cleansed and nourished at the same time. One can be confident of complete safety and real health-building results.

To prepare for the wheat grass fast, it is essential for the patient to undertake repeated warm water enema so as to cleanse the body of accumulated waste products. It is necessary to eliminate this putrefaction. The wheat grass fast consists of three or four wheat grass juice drinks each day plus two chlorophyll implants. If the patient does not like the taste or odour of the juice, he can take four implants instead of two, with same beneficial results.

Upon awakening, the patient should drink two glasses of warm water, mixed with the juice of one lemon and sweetened with molasses or honey. Then, the colon should be thoroughly evacuated with an enema to eliminate any debris clogging to the inner walls of the colon. The patient should sip 120 ml of pure wheat grass chlorophyll three times a day at five-hourly intervals. Each drink may be diluted with water on 50:50 basis. While on wheat grass therapy, the patient should drink at least one litre of not-too-cold water each day, placing a small bunch of wheat-grass in each drink to purify it.

CHAPTER 12

CARMINATIVE FOODS

Herbs and spices have long been used in ancient medicine as carminatives—agents that help expel gas and relief flatulence. The main pharmacological agent is considered to be oils in the plants. These oils relax smooth muscles, thereby allowing gas to escape. In some cases the gas erupts upward through a relaxed sphincter muscle between the esophagus and the stomach. Then it is called a burp or a belch. Carminatives also have an antispasmodic, muscle-relaxing effect in the intestine.

FOODS THAT RELIEVE GAS

Alfalfa, Aniseed, Asafoetida, Bishop's Weed, Butter Milk, Caraway Seeds, Chamomile, Chebulic Myroblan, Cinnamon, Citrus Fruits, Clove, Coconut, Dill, Fennel Seeds, Garlic, Ginger, Mint, Parsley and Pumpkin.

Alfalfa

The seeds of alfalfa, known as 'King of sprouts', are of immense value in the maintenance of health. Their daily use can help build up immunity to stomach distress. Alfalfa, in the form of herb tea, provides vital alkalizing benefits for hyperacid stomach and helps prevent gas formation and relieves accumulated gas. It tends to control the flow of hydrochloric acid and aids the action of gastric enzyme,

135

pepsin. The addition of mint to alfalfa tea helps settle disturbed stomach after a sumptuous meal.

Aniseed

This spice possesses gas-relieving property. It is an excellent medicine for expelling wind from the stomach. It can also be taken, in combination with other digestive foods like ginger, cumin and pepper, in the form of an infusion.

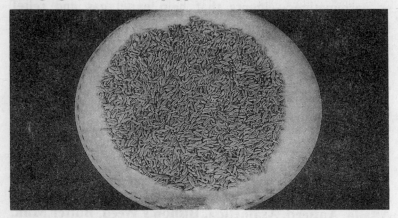

Aniseed possesses gas-relieving property and is an excellent medicine for expelling wind from the stomach.

An easy way to prepare the infusion is to mix a teaspoon of aniseed in a cup of boiling water and leave it covered overnight. The clear fluid is then decanted and taken with honey. This helps gurgling in the abdomen. This is also useful in preventing gas and fermentation in the stomach and the bowels.

Asafoetida

Asafoetida is a resinous gum of a tall perennial plant, with robust carrot-shaped roots. It is dirty yellow in colour with a pungent smell. It is used as a flavouring agent and forms a constituent of many spice mixtures.

Asafoetida is an anti flatulent food. It is an ideal medicine for several stomach disorders. It is one of the best remedies for expelling wind from the stomach. This spice is an ingredient for most of the digestive powders. In case of flatulence and distension of the stomach, Asafoetida should be dissolved in hot water and a pad of cloth steeped in it and used for fomenting the abdomen.

Bishop's Weed

Bishop's weed has long been used in indigenous medicine for the treatment of various digestive disorders including flatulence and indigestion. For expelling gas from the stomach, the seeds may be eaten with betel leaves. A teaspoon of these seeds with a little rock salt is a household remedy for indigestion and gas formation.

The volatile oil extracted from the seeds is also useful in indigestion and gas formation. It is usually given in doses of 1 to 3 drops. *Omum* water, that is, the water distilled from the seeds, is an excellent remedy for flatulent dyspepsia.

In case of flatulence, bishop's weed and dried ginger in equal weight may be soaked in two-and-half times the quantity of limejuice. This mixture should than be dried and powdered with a little black salt. About two grams of this powder should be taken with warm water in treating this condition.

Butter milk

Thin buttermilk is a very simple and effective remedy for relieving gas in the stomach. It should be mixed with a quarter teaspoon of pepper powder. For better results, an equal quantity of cumin powder may be added to the buttermilk. Buttermilk enema is also highly beneficial in expelling gas from the stomach.

Caraway Seeds

The caraway seeds are a popular spice and a flavouring agent. The dried fruits or seeds are brown in colour, hard and sharp to touch. They have pleasant odour, aromatic flavour, sharp taste and leave somewhat warm feeling in the mouth.

Caraway seeds are a food of great value for relieving gas in the stomach. They expel wind from the stomach and are useful in flatulent colic, countering any possible adverse effects of medicines. However, the volatile oil of the seeds is used more often than the seeds themselves. For flatulence, a cup of tea made from caraway seeds taken thrice a day, after meals, will give relief. This tea is prepared by adding a teaspoon of caraway seeds in 1.5 to 2 litres of boiling water and allowing them to simmer on a slow fire for 15 minutes. The water is then strained and sipped hot or warm.

Chamomile

Chamomile, also known as bitter or German chamomile, is a popular herb. It is an erect annual plant. The flowers of this plant constitute the drug chamomile. They contain many medicinal virtues. They relieve flatulence and induce copious perspiration. They are also stimulants.

Chamomile possesses anti-gas activity. It expels wind from the stomach and is an effective remedy for digestive disorders, especially of nervous origin. It can be used beneficially in dyspepsia, flatulence and colic. A powder of the flowers or one to three drops of oil extracted from flowers is taken in 1 to 2 gram doses in the treatment of these disorders.

Chebulic Myroblan

Chebulic myroblan is a carminative food. It helps relieve gas in the stomach. Its juice is very valuable in the treatment of acidity and heart-burn. It neutralises too much acidity in the stomach, if taken after principal meals. For better results, this juice should be combined with the juice of Indian gooseberry. Chewing a piece of chebulic myroblan is an age-old remedy for heartburn.

Cinnamon

Cinnamon stimulates digestion and relieves gas in the stomach. Coarsely powdered and boiled in a glass of water with a pinch of pepper powder and honey, it can be beneficially used as a carminative medicine for flatulence and indigestion. A tablespoon of this water should be taken half an hour after meals.

Citrus Fruit

The term citrus fruit includes orange, lemon, grapefruit, lime, malta and mosambi. They play an important role in building health. In addition to being one of the most valuable sources of vitamin C in the diet, they are valuable for their tartness and flavour.

The value of citrus fruits emanate from large amounts of vitamin C, calcium and oligo elements, as well as from easily assimilated sugars, citric acid and citrates contained in them. These substances play a vital role in the body's activities.

The citrus fruits are fairly acidic to taste, but when they are burnt in the tissues, they leave an alkaline residue, so that their ultimate effect is to maintain the normal alkaline reserve of the body. Their acids do not increase the body's acidity, but in fact have opposite effect. Acid salts of organic acids, such as potassium citrate, lose their original acidity by oxidation. Thus, all that is left are alkaline elements.

All citrus fruits are thus gas relieving foods and are highly beneficial in the treatment of hyperacidity, indigestion and other digestive disorders. The most important of these fruits are lemon and lime. Lemon juice reaches the stomach and attacks the bacteria, inhibiting the formation of acids. Limejuice also acts in the similar way. A teaspoon of fresh limejuice, mixed with equal quantity of honey, and licked, will help stop bilious vomiting, indigestion, burning in the chest and excessive accumulation of saliva in the mouth. A teaspoon of limejuice mixed with water and a pinch of soda-bicarb makes an excellent remedy for acidity in the stomach. It also acts as a powerful carminative in case of indigestion.

Clove

This popular spice is of great value as a gas relieving food. It is highly beneficial in the treatment of several digestive disorders like indigestion and flatulent colic. A decoction should be prepared by boiling 6 cloves in 30 ml of water. This decoction should be taken thrice daily after meals as a carminative medicine in treating these conditions.

Coconut

Coconut Water is a carminative food of great value. It is an excellent remedy for gas formation and heartburn. It gives the stomach necessary rest and provides vitamins and minerals. The stomach is greatly helped in coming back to normal condition, if nothing else except coconut water is taken during the first 24 hours.

The mature, dried coconut is also a good remedy for acidity. The oil of the coconut reduces the acid secretion of the stomach and gives much relief to the patient.

Cucumber

This popular vegetable fruit helps greatly in relieving acidity and gas in the stomach. The juice of the cucumber is a medicine par excellence for hyperacidity and gastric ulcer. It gives immediate relief to the burning sensation in the stomach. This juice should be given to the patient every two hours in doses of 120ml to 180ml, at a time, in treating these conditions. As the cucumber is about 96 per cent water, sufficient juice can be easily extracted from it.

Dill

Dill is a valuable carminative food. Its oil, obtained by distillation of the seeds, is an effective medicine for hyperacidity and flatulent colic. A drop of dill oil given with castor oil prevents gripping pain in the abdomen and increases its purgative action by relaxing the intestines.

Fennel Seeds

Fennel seeds are a valuable food for relieving gas and removing wind from the stomach. An infusion is prepared by boiling a tablespoon of fennel seeds in 100 ml of water for half an hour. This infusion is highly beneficial in the treatment of indigestion, biliousness and flatulence.

Garlic

Garlic is reputed in folk medicine as an anti-flatulent food of great importance. Adding a little garlic while cooking beans or other gaseous vegetables takes away their harmful gas-forming properties. Recent studies at G. B. Pant University in India have shown its effectiveness as a carminative food. After discovering green peas to be a major producer of gas in animals in experiments, the investigators did a test on dogs by adding a little garlic, amounts generally used in cooking, to the peas. They found garlic to be preventive against gas formation. It took away nearly all the gas-producing power out of peas. When the dogs got peas with garlic, gas production was no greater than it was from a wheat cereal, which was the least gaseous food tested.

Ginger

Ancient physicians used ginger as a carminative and anti-fermenting medicine. Taken internally, it is a stimulating carminative. It is a valuable drug in flatulence. Chewing a fresh piece of ginger after meals regularly is an insurance against these ailments. This protective action is attributable to excessive secretion of saliva, diastase enzyme and volatile oil. A hot drink made by infusing a small quantity of powdered or root ginger makes an excellent carminative. It should be taken after meals and should always be slowly sipped.

Mint

Mint is a popular spice, used extensively in Indian cooking. It contains plenty of vitamins and is rich in several minerals. It is much valued as a stimulant and as a drug that relieves flatulence. It is useful in strengthening the stomach and promoting its action and also in counteracting spasmodic disorders.

Mint possesses anti-gas property. The juice extracted from the leaves is a good appetiser. Its value is greatly enhanced

Mint is a carminative food and helps relieve gas in the stomach.

by mixing an equal amount of honey and lemon juice to it. This mixture forms a very effective remedy for indigestion and gaseous distension of the stomach.

Parsley

Parsley aids digestion and helps prevent the formation of gas in the stomach and intestines. It is one of the most popular remedies for indigestion and flatulence. A couple of sprigs of the fresh vegetable or a quarter teaspoon of the dried vegetable should be taken with a glass of water in treating these conditions. As, however, fresh parsley is sometimes rather tough, it should be well masticated.

Pumpkin

The pumpkin is an alkaline food and a mild laxative. It is easily digested and non-gas forming. Its juice has been found to be very effective in relieving discomforts in the digestive system due to excessive acidity. For acute stomach pains due to hyperacidity and indigestion, about 120 ml. of diluted juice should be used. This juice can be prepared by grinding the pulp with water and strained through a thin cloth. It can be mixed with honey and fresh limejuice before use.

CHAPTER 13

CHOLESTEROL LOWERING FOODS

Cholesterol is a yellow fatty substance and a principal ingredient in the digestive juice bile, in the fatty sheaths that insulate nerves and in sex hormones, namely estrogen and androgen. It performs several functions such as transportation of fat, providing defense mechanism, protecting red blood cells and muscular membrane of the body.

Most of the cholesterol found in the body is produced in the liver. However, about 20 to 30 per cent generally come from the foods we eat. Some cholesterol is also secreted into the intestinal tract in bile and gets mixed with the dietary cholesterol. The percentage of ingested cholesterol absorbed seems to average 40 to 50 per cent of the intake. In blood, cholesterol is bound with certain proteins-lipoproteins, which have an affinity for blood fats, known as lipids. There are two main types of lipoproteins, a low density one (LDL) and a high density one (HDL). The low-density lipoprotein is the one, which is considered harmful and is associated with cholesterol deposits in blood vessels. The higher the ratio of LDL to the total cholesterol, the greater will be the risk of arterial damage and heart disease. The HDL on the other hand plays a beneficial role by helping remove cholesterol from circulation and thereby reduce the risk of heart disease.

Foods can lower bad-type LDL cholesterol, raise good-type HDL cholesterol and help prevent the oxidation of LDL cholesterol that makes it more destructive to arteries. On the other hand, some foods, such as oats, are considered to reduce supplies of bile acids in the intestinal tract that otherwise would turn into cholesterol. Food antioxidants may also help keep bad-type LDL cholesterol from becoming oxidised and toxic to arteries.

Several years ago, scientists at the U.S Department of Agriculture's laboratory at the University of Wisconsin in Madison, discovered that food substances called tocotrienols suppress an enzyme that hampers the liver's manufacture of cholesterol. Cells needing cholesterol then suck it out of the bloodstream and cholesterol blood levels go down.

Other foods create different chemicals that seem also to turn down internal cholesterol production. That is precisely how the potent cholesterol-reducing drug Mevacor (lovastatin) also works.

FOODS THAT LOWER LDL CHOLESTEROL

Almond, Apple, Avocado, Beans (dried), Carrot, Coriander seeds (dried), Fenugreek Seeds, Garlic, Grapefruit, Grape Seed Oil, Ishabgul, Oats, Olive Oil, Onion, Safflower Oil, Soyabeans, Sunflower Seeds and Walnuts.

Almond

Almond, the most important of all nuts, is a highly nutritious food. It is high in monounsaturated fat, which is known to reduce cholesterol. In a research study, Dr. Gene Spiller made men and women with fairly high cholesterol, averaging around 6.24,eat 100grams of almonds a day for three to nine weeks. Others ate equal amounts of fat from cheese or olive oil. The average cholesterol of the almond eaters came down 10 to 15 per cent compared to that of the cheese eaters. Almonds and olive oil exercised beneficial effects, as most of the fat contained in both is chemically identical.

Apple

Apple, with its high soluble fibre called pectin, can help lower cholesterol. In a recent research, French scientists had a group of middle-aged healthy men and women add two or three apples a day to their ordinary diet for a month. LDL cholesterol fell in 80 per cent of them, and by more than 10 per cent in half of them. Good type HDL Cholesterol also went up. Interestingly, the apples benefited women more than men. One woman's cholesterol came down by 30 per cent.

In another study, David Gee, Ph.D. at Central Washington University tested high-fibre apple waste left over from making apple juice. He had the apple fibre baked into cookies. When 26 men with fairly high cholesterol ate three apple cookies a day, instead of a placebo cookie, their cholesterol came down by seven per cent on an average. Each apple cookie had 15grams of fibre, equal to the amount in four or five apples, he says.

Most experts attribute cholesterol lowering quality in apple to pectin contained in it, although other components in this fruit also help lower cholesterol. As Dr. David Kritchevsky of the Wistar Institute in Philadelphia points out, a whole apple lowers cholesterol more than its pectin content predicts. "Something else is at work also", he says.

Avocado

Avocado is a valuable cholesterol lowering food. It has rich concentrations of the same type cholesterol lowering fat as almonds and olive oil. Research scientists in Israil found that eating avocados, as well as almonds and olive oil for three months, cut detrimental LDL cholesterol by about 12 per cent in a group of men.

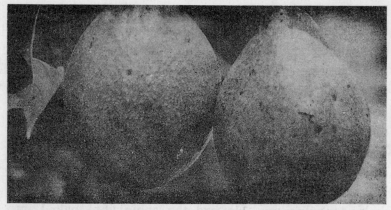

Avocado, with its beneficial fats, is a valuable cholesterol lowering food.

Australian cardiologists at the Wesley Medical Centre in Queensland also found recently that eating one half to one and a half avocados a day is more effective in reducing cholesterol than low-fat diet. In the test conducted by them, 15 women ate a high-carbohydrate, low-fat diet with 20 per cent fat calories and an avocado high-fat diet with 37 per cent fat calories, each for three weeks. The raw avocados were put in salads or spread on bread or crackers. The result was that average cholesterol came down by 4.9 per cent on the low-fat diet compared with nearly twice as much that is 8.2 per cent, on the avocado diet.

Moreover, the low-fat diet also lowered good HDL

cholesterol by as much as 14 per cent, but did not lower bad LDL cholesterol. Very-low-fat diets often do this. On the other hand, the avocados attacked only detrimental LDL cholesterol. Investigators noted that avocados also protected arteries against oxidative damage that makes cholesterol dangerous.

Beans (dried)

Beans or legumes are one of the fastest-acting and safest cholesterol lowering foods. Studies show that they consistently help lower cholesterol. According to James Anderson, M.D., of the University of Kentucky College of Medicine, eating 170 grams of cooked dried beans a day generally reduces bad cholesterol by about 20 per cent. The result can be expected in about three weeks. All types of bean are valuable in this respect. About 170 grams of dried or 340 grams of baked beans a day also raise good type HDL cholesterol by about nine per cent. This does not happen immediately, but usually after a year or two. According to one test, beans improve the HDL-LDL cholesterol ratio by 17 per cent. Dr. Anderson advises an intake of 85 grams of beans each at lunch and dinner to obtain best results. Beans contain at least six cholesterol-reducing compounds, the most important of which is soluble fibre.

Carrot

This vegetable helps lower bad LDL cholesterol and raise good HDL cholesterol. According to Dr. Philip Pfeffer, Ph. D., and Peter Hoagland, Ph.D., scientists at the U.S. Department of Agriculture's Eastern Regional Research Centre, carrots contain high anti-cholesterol soluble fibre including pectin. Dr. Pfeffer calculates that the fibre in a couple of carrots a day can lower cholesterol by 10-20 per cent, which would bring many people with moderately high cholesterol into the normal range. After he started eating a couple of carrots a day, his own blood cholesterol came down by about 20 per cent.

A test carried out in Canada discovered that men who ate about two and a half carrots every day found that their cholesterol level came down by 11 per cent on an average. According to a German study, the amount of beta-carotene in one or two carrots also raised good HDL cholesterol significantly. The carrot fibre continues to have medicinal properties whether the vegetable is eaten raw, cooked, frozen, canned or in liquid form says Dr. Pfeffer.

Coriander Seeds (dried)

The seeds of coriander are a popular spice used extensively in Indian cooking. The seeds are dried when they are ripe. They have an aromatic odour and agreeable spicy taste. These seeds possess cholesterol lowering property. Their use has thus been found beneficial in the treatment of high blood cholesterol. A decoction should be prepared by boiling two tablespoons of dry seeds in a glass of water. It should be cooled and strained. This decoction should be taken twice daily for few months to bring down blood cholesterol level.

Fenugreek Seeds

The scientists all over the world are discovering the medicinal benefits of Fenugreek seeds. Daniel Mowrey of the American Phytotherapy Research Laboratory in Salt Lake City, Utah, firmly believes that they reduce cholesterol. The seeds also help reduce sugar levels in non-insulin dependent diabetics.

Indian researchers have done significant work on Fenugreek and its medicinal properties. According to research studies conducted at National Institute of Nutrition, Hyderabad, fenugreek seeds were given in varying doses of 25 grams to 100 grams daily, to diabetes patients. Besides reducing their levels of glucose, the seeds also reduced serum cholesterol and tryglycerides in them. The seeds can be used as an infusion, or in the form of tea.

Israeli scientists at Hebrew University of Jerusalem also have shown that fenugreek seeds can lower blood sugar and cholesterol in both diabetics and healthy people. Additionally, they have identified an active ingredient in fenugreek seeds. It is a gel-like soluble fibre called galacto-mannan. In animal studies, the fenugreek gel binds up bile acids, lowering cholesterol, much the same way as common drugs do.

Garlic

Garlic is of great value as a cholesterol lowering food. The use of garlic has been found highly beneficial in treatment of high blood cholesterol. About 20 published human tests show that fresh garlic and some garlic preparations reduce cholesterol substantially. According to Robert Lin, Ph.D., Chairman of a recent international conference on the health aspects of garlic, three fresh garlic cloves a day can lower cholesterol by 10 per cent on an average and up to 15 per cent in some cases. It does not matter whether the garlic is cooked or raw, he says. It is effective both ways. Six compounds in garlic have been identified that lower cholesterol by reducing liver's synthesis of cholesterol.

of cholesterol.

In a recent test, at L.T.M. Medical College in Bombay, 50 persons ate three raw garlic cloves every morning for two months. Their cholesterol came down by 15 per cent from an average 5.54 to 4.68. Their blood clotting factors also improved dramatically. In another study, at Bastyr College in Seattle, a daily dose of garlic oil from three fresh garlic cloves brought cholesterol down seven per cent in a month, but, more important, raised good-type HDL by 23 per cent.

The researchers, Dr. Christopher Silagy and Dr. Andrew Neil of Oxford University, also conducted trials about garlic's power in lowering cholesterol. They found on an average, a 12 per cent reduction in cholesterol, evident after one month. Best results were obtained from the trials lasting at least three months. The typical dose was an equivalent of 600 to 900mg of garlic powder. Garlic powder, fresh garlic, garlic extract and garlic oil were all used in the various trials.

Grapefruit

The pulp of grapefruit, the segments with membranes and tiny juice sacs, contain a unique type of soluble fibre called galacturonic acid that helps lower blood cholesterol. It also helps dissolve plaque or reverse plaque formaiton already clogging the arteries. In one study by Dr. James Cerda, professor of gastroenterology at the University of Florida, it was discovered that the grapefruit fibre, found in about 340g of grapefruit segments eaten every day, lowered blood cholesterol by about 10 per cent. It may be clarified that the juice of this fruit does not contain fibre or show any cholesterol lowering effects. Furthermore, in studies on pigs, which have cardiovascular systems similar to human beings, Dr. Cerda noted that the grapefruit compound actually resulted in less diseased and narrowed arteries and aorta. These compounds somehow swept away some of the built-up plaque.

Grape Seed Oil

The oil extracted from grape seed, which is used for a mild dressing, is a valuable food for raising good HDL cholesterol. David T. Nash, a cardiologist at the State University of New York Health Science Center in Syracuse, tested grape seed oil on 23 men and women who had low HDL — below 1.17. Every day for four weeks, they ate two tablespoons of grape seed oil in addition to their regular low-fat diet. Their HDL cholesterol increased by an average 14 per cent. Dr. Nash said that some did not respond, but HDL cholesterol did go up in more than half of them. Generally, those who already had the highest HDL cholesterol were unlikely to get further increase from the grape seed oil.

Ishabgul

The seeds of this popular herb contain blood cholesterol lowering property. Their use has been found beneficial in the treatment of high blood cholesterol. The oil of the seeds should be used for this purpose. This oil contains 50 per cent linoleic acid and is more active than even sunflower oil. One teaspoon of this oil should be taken twice daily to achieve beneficial results.

Oats

Eating oats lowers blood cholesterol. Dutch scientists discovered the anti-cholesterol power of oats four decades ago. This has now been confirmed by 23 out of 25 studies, says Michael C. Davidson, M.D., Assistant Professor of Cardiology at Rush-Presbyterian-St. Luke's Medical Center in Chicago.

Dr. Davidson reported in a recent study that a medium-sized bowl of cooked oat bran or a large bowl of oatmeal can help lower blood cholesterol. According to him, the biggest dose a person can have is 55 grams of oat bran a day. This amount reduced detrimental cholesterol 16 per cent in those eating a low-fat diet. Half of that would cut cholesterol 10 per cent. However, taking in 85 grams of oat bran daily did not lower cholesterol further. Oatmeal can also serve the same purpose but it has to be taken in double the quantity of oat bran for the same impact.

Olive Oil

Olive oil, being high in monounsaturated fats, is a food of great value as an artery protector that lowers bad LDL cholesterol, without lowering good HDL cholesterol. It also keeps LDL cholesterol safe from toxic changes that threaten arteries and promote heart attacks. A remarkable research study even discovered that olive oil was superior to the standard low-fat diet recommended for reducing cholesterol. In this study subjects were made to eat 41 per cent of their calories in fat, most of it from olive oil. Their bad LDL cholesterol fell more than when they ate a diet with half as much fat. It was also found that good HDL cholesterol increased on the olive oil diet but decreased on low-fat diet.

In another research study, Dr. Daniel Steinberg of University of California, found that olive oil dramatically prevents toxic oxidation of LDL cholesterol. In this study Dr. Steinberg and colleagues gave one group of healthy persons about 40 per cent of their daily intake of calories, in monounsaturated fat, equal to about 3 tablespoons of olive oil a day. Others were given regular safflower oil low in monounsaturated fatty acids. Then researchers examined the bad-type LDL cholesterol from both groups. They found that LDL cholesterol of the monounsaturated oil eaters was only half as likely to become oxidised and thus be able to clog arteries. This suggests that when a person eats fat, the olive oil monounsaturated type is a good choice to forestall artery clogging.

Onion

Onions are credited with the property to lower bad LDL cholesterol and raise good HDL type. Raw onion is one of the best treatments for boosting beneficial HDL cholesterol. According to Dr. Victor Gurewich, a cardiologist and professor of medicine at Harvard Medical School, half a raw onion, or equivalent in juice, raises HDL an average 30 per cent in most people with heart disease or cholesterol problems. Based on folklore tradition about the use of onion as medicine, he tested it in his clinic. The test proved very successful. So, he advises all his patients to eat onions. He, however, says that more you cook the onions, the more they lose their HDL-raising powers. The onion therapy works in about 70 per cent of patients. If a person cannot eat half a raw onion a day, he may eat less. Any amount may help raise good HDL cholesterol.

Safflower Oil

Safflower oil is a food of exceptional value in lowering blood cholesterol. It possesses the highest linoleic acid content of all edible oils, being 72 per cent on an average. It is one of the most polyunsaturated. The medicinal value of linoleic acid came into prominence in the 1960s following the publication in a series of medical and scientific journals, the findings of researchers. These findings proved that this fatty acid was highly beneficial in lowering serum cholesterol levels in laboratory animals and humans. From virtual obscurity, safflower oil became a best seller within a few years.

Soyabeans

Soyabeans are one of the best foods to lower cholesterol. This is attributable to its richness in lecithin. Lecithin, is a fatty food substance and is the most abundant of the phospholipids. This substance is highly beneficial in case of increase in cholesterol level. It has the ability to break up cholesterol into small particles, which can be easily handled by the system.

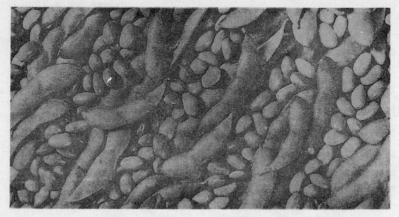

Soyabeans, as a rich source of lecithin, are one of the
best foods to lower cholesterol.

With sufficient intake of lecithin, cholesterol cannot build up against the walls of the arteries and veins. It also increases the production of bile acids made from cholesterol, thereby reducing its amount in the blood. Other good vegetarian food sources of lecithin are vegetable oils, whole grain cereals and unpasteurised milk.

Sunflower Seeds

Sunflower seeds are probably the most familiar of all edible seeds. They are the tightly packed core of the splendid sunflowers. Sunflower kernels are well above average in protein, phosphorus and iron concentration. They are very rich sources of B-complex vitamins.

Sunflower seeds are cholesterol lowering food. The seeds contain substantial quantity of linoleic acid, which is the fat helpful in reducing cholesterol deposits on the walls of arteries. Substituting sunflower seeds for some of the solid fats like butter and cream will therefore, help control blood cholesterol and also lead to great improvement in health.

Walnut

This popular nut is also a food of great value in lowering blood cholesterol. This has been brought out by latest research conducted by Dr. Joan Sabate of Loma Linda University. She studied persons with normal blood cholesterol. All were on a low-fat diet, but for one month they ate 20 per cent of their calories in walnuts, about 55g of walnuts in a daily 1,800-calorie diet. For another month, they ate no nuts. On the no-nuts diet, their cholesterol dropped an average 6 per cent but on the walnut-eating regime, their cholesterol fell 18 per cent. Average cholesterol dropped 0.57 points. Thus, walnuts added a cholesterol-reducing substance even to an ordinary low-fat diet.

CHAPTER 14

DIURETIC FOODS

Some foods serve as diuretics. However, plant foods do not function as diuretics the same way as do the pharmaceutical drugs. This opinion has been expressed by plant expert Dr. Varro Tyler of Purdue University. Pharmaceutical diuretics increase the excretion of water and salt, whereas plant foods stimulate only a loss of water and not sodium. They should therefore be appropriately called "aquaretics", says Dr. Tyler. These foods do this by irritating the cellular filters of the kidneys. However, their irritating mechanism could be detrimental to those having kidney disease. Such persons should therefore avoid the use of diuretic foods.

FOODS THAT INCREASE SECRETION OF URINE

Alfalfa, Banana Stem, Barley, Betel Leaf, Bottle Gourd, Cardamom, Coconut, Cucumber, Dandelion, Drumstick Flower, Grapes, Honey, Ladies finger, Musk Melon, Onion, Orange, Parslane, Parsley, Radish, Spinach, Sugarcane and Watermelon.

Alfalfa

Alfalfa contains several of the digestive enzymes, and carries nearly two per cent chlorophyll, which is about the richest of all plants. This green and wonder-working substance, in addition to its healing properties, has been found to be slightly laxative, digestive, diuretic and a splendid tonic. Being a good diuretic, it acts gently upon the kidneys. Many doctors have used it successfully for dropsy and inflammation of the bladder.

Alfalfa can be used in the form of juice extracted from leaves or in the form of herb tea, which is made from seeds as well as from dried leaves of the plant. The tea from seeds is prepared by cooking them in an enamel pan with the lid on for half an hour. After cooking, it should be strained, squeezing or pressing seeds dry. It should be allowed to cool after adding honey to taste and put in a refrigerator. Cold or hot water should be added to taste before use.

Banana stem

Fresh juice from the porous stem of banana tree is an excellent diuretic food. It is rich in potassium, vitamins and other minerals. A glassful of this juice taken early in the morning acts as a very powerful diuretic in all conditions where profuse urination is indicated.

Barley

Barley possesses diuretic property. It should be used in the form of gruel for this purpose. Its gruel, especially in combination with buttermilk and limejuice, makes a valuable diuretic carbohydrate food. This combination is highly beneficial in the treatment of urinary disorders like nephritis and bladder infection.

Betel Leaf

The betel leaves are credited with diuretic properties. The juice should be extracted from these leaves and mixed with dilute milk and sweetened slightly. This mixture makes an excellent diuretic, which increases the secretion and discharge of urine. It is a specific medicine for scanty urination.

Bottle gourd

This popular vegetable is of great value as a diuretic food. It is very effective in urinary disorders. A glass of fresh juice prepared by grating the whole fruit should be mixed with a teaspoon of limejuice. It should be taken once daily in the treatment of burning sensation in urinary passage due to high acidity of urine. It should be taken with sulpha drugs in the treatment of urinary infection. It acts as an alkaline diuretic in this condition.

Cardamom

Cardamom helps increase the secretion and discharge of urine. Its powdered seeds, mixed with a tablespoon of banana leaf and Indian goosebery juice, taken thrice a day, serve as a valuable diuretic food. It is very effective in treating diseases like gonorrhoea, cystitis, nephritis, burning micturition or urination and scanty urination.

Coconut

The coconut water is a very effective diuretic food. It contains a very high concentration of potassium and chlorine in sterilized water. It is of exceptional value in urinary disorders. It acts as a natural diuretic in heart, liver and kidney disorders such as scanty and suppressed urination, albuminuria, dropsy, high acidity of urine and gonorrhoea. It is one of the cheapest food diuretics that protect from the bad effects of excessive use of oral chlorothiazide diuretics. In case of kidney failure, coconut water should be very carefully given under the strict supervision of a physician.

Cucumber

Cucumber is one of the most important diuretic foods. Its juice has been found very effective in treating urinary system disorders like bladder infection, nephritis and scanty urination. A glass of this juice should be taken twice daily mixed with two teaspoons of honey and a teaspoon of limejuice. It will act as a powerful diuretic in the treatment of these diseases.

Dandelion

Dandelion is a hardy perennial herb and a tasty salad vegetable. It has a remarkable nutritional value. It contains almost as much iron as spinach, four times the vitamin A content of lettuce and is a very rich source of magnesium, potassium, vitamin C, calcium and sodium. It also contains protein, fat and carbohydrates.

Dandelion is a diuretic food. It increases secretion and discharge of urine. Tea made from its buds, flowers, fresh leaves or even blanched leaves, can be beneficially used in urinary disorders like retention of urine and slow start to pass urine. It is essential to drink lots of water and other harmless drinks with this treatment.

Tender leaves of dandelion can be used as a salad vegetable. They can also be cooked in a little boiling water or in combination with spinach and cooked in the same way. Soup can also be made with chopped dandelion leaves. The dried leaves are used for tea and as an ingredient in diet drinks.

Drumstick Flower

The drumstick is a fairly common vegetable grown all over India. It is valued mainly for the tender pod. It is antibacterial and a wonderful cleanser. The flowers of drumstick tree are a diuretic food. Fresh juice should be extracted from these flowers. A teaspoon of this juice, mixed with half a glass of tender coconut water, makes an excellent diuretic medicine and can be taken twice daily in treating conditions like bladder infection with beneficial results.

Grapes

The grape has an exceptional diuretic value on account of its high contents of water and potassium salt. Its low albumin and sodium chloride contents enhance its value in urinary system disorder. It is an excellent food in acute and chronic nephritis and in kidney and bladder stones.

Honey

Honey is a valuable diuretic food. It contains mineral salts and is hence endowed with unique properties to facilitate profuse urination. It is a very effective remedy for retention of urine. About 70 grams of honey should be taken mixed with 4 grams of sugar in treating this condition. It acts as a powerful diuretic and urination will start immediately.

Lady's Finger

The lady's finger is a very popular table vegetable grown all over India. It contains a large quantity of bland, viscid, mucilage, which is valuable in allaying irritation of the skin. It exercises a soothing effect on the skin and mucous membranes.

A decoction made from lady's finger forms an effective

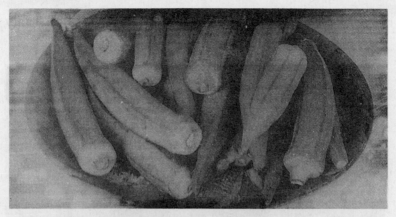

A decoction made from Lady's finger is an effective diuretic food.

diuretic food. This decoction is prepared by boiling 90 grams of the fresh capsules, cut transversely, in half a litre of water for 20 minutes and then strained and sweetened. It can be given with beneficial result in doses of 60 to 90 ml. frequently, in all irritable condition of genito-urinary organs, such as dysuria, gonorrhoea and leucorrhoea and in all cases attendant with scalding, pain and difficulty in passing urine.

Musk Melon

The musk melon occupies a place of pride among the summer delicacies. The fruit is called musk melon from the musk-like odour it emits. The ripe melon is highly nourishing. The seeds of this fruit yield sweet edible oil, which is nutritive and diuretic.

This fruit is a valuable diuretic food. A quarter Kg. of this fruit should be used for the purpose in summer and a piece of sugarcandy sucked after its use. The regular use of musk melon 3 or 4 times daily causes profuse micturition. The use of water should be restricted with this treatment. It may be replaced by slightly sweetened milk. The pulp of the fruit being a powerful diuretic is highly useful in cases of scanty or suppressed urination.

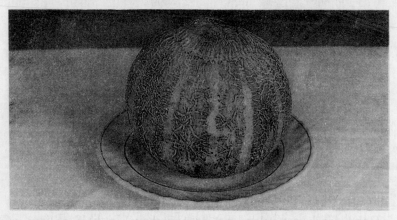

The use of musk melon promotes secretion and discharge of urine.

In Ayurveda, the rind of melon is regarded as a sure cure for urine retention. Melon rind is rubbed in water and the strained water is given to the patient in summer. In the winter season, it is warmed slightly before administration. This will promote clear micturition.

Onion

Onion is an effective diuretic food and very beneficial in the treatment of urinary system disorders. For burning sensation with micturition, a decoction of this vegetable has proved very valuable. This decoction is prepared by boiling 6g of onions in 500 ml of water. It should be removed from the fire when half of the water has evaporated. It should then be strained and taken by the patient when cool.

In retention of urine, onion should be rubbed in water and 60 grams of sugar should be mixed with it. The patient should take this mixture and it will result in free urination within a short time. The effect will be greatly enhanced if a little potassium nitrate is added to this mixture.

Orange

The juice of orange is an effective diuretic food when mixed with tender coconut water. It serves as a natural diuretic in all cases of scanty urination, dropsy, nephritis, cystitis, gonorrhoeal, non-specific urethritis and painful micturition due to high acidity of the urine.

Parslane

This green leafy vegetable is a diuretic food. It increases the secretion and discharge of urine. It is thus a valuable diet in dysuria, which is marked by pain or difficulty in passing urine. A teaspoon of the infusion of the leaves should be given twice daily in treating this condition. The seeds of this vegetable are also useful in treating scanty urination due to excessive sweating. An emulsion, prepared by mixing a teaspoon of the seeds in a glass of tender coconut water can cure these disorders. This emulsion should be administered thrice daily. It also reduces burning sensation in bladder infection.

Parsley

Parsley possesses diuretic properties. It is an aquaretic food, which stimulates loss of water, says Dr. Varro Tyler. According to him, drinking parsley tea is a very effective way to stimulate loss of water. This tea can be prepared by putting a couple of teaspoons of dried parsley in a cup of boiling water. It increases the secretion and discharge of urine. According to R.D. Pope, M.D, who has done considerable research on the subject, parsley is excellent for the genito-urinary tract. It is of great assistance in the calculii of the kidneys and bladder, albuminuria, nephritis and other kidney troubles.

Radish

The leaves and tape roots of radish are diuretic foods, which increase the secretion and discharge of urine. A cup of radish leaf juice given once daily for a fortnight, acts as a curative medicine in dissolving gravel in urinary tract and cystitis, which is marked by inflammation of urinary bladder. This juice is also useful in cases of difficulty in passing urine (dysuria), passing of urine in painful drops (stranguary) and in urinary and syphilitic complaints. This juice may be given in doses mentioned above and repeated as often as necessary.

Spinach

The leaves of spinach are an effective diuretic food. They increase the secretion and discharge of urine. Fresh spinach juice, taken with tender coconut water once or twice a day, acts as a very effective but safe diuretic due to the combined action of both nitrates and potassium. It can be safely given in bladder infection, nephritis and scanty urination due to dehydration.

Sugarcane

Sugarcane is the most important member of the plant kingdom with a metabolism leading to the accumulation of sucrose. It is transported as glucose and fructose within the growing plant. The crop provides the cheapest form of energy- giving food. The juice is nutritious and refreshing. It contains about 15 per cent natural sugar and is rich in organic salts and vitamins.

The juice of sugarcane is a very effective diuretic food. It is highly beneficial in scanty urination. It keeps the urinary flow clear and helps the kidneys perform their functions properly. It is also valuable in burning micturition due to high acidity, gonorrhoea, enlarged prostate, cystitis and nephritis. For better results, it should be mixed with limejuice, ginger juice and coconut water.

Watermelon

Watermelon contains the highest concentration of water amongst all the fruits. It is also rich in potassium salts and has a base forming property. It is thus one of the safest and best diuretics, which can be used with beneficial results in scanty urination, kidney and bladder stones and excess discharge of phosphates in the urine. It is also valuable in affections of the urinary organs like gonorrhea. The pulp may be rejected when it is to be consumed in large quantities as the entire food Value is contained in the juice.

CHAPTER 15

<u>IMMUNITY STIMULATING FOODS</u>

Immune system is a complex interaction among cells in many parts of the body. They all co-ordinate to protect the body from foreign invaders. The immune system is not located in any one organ system or part of the body. The brain, the blood, the liver, the bone marrow, the lymph system, the spleen, the thymus, the skin, and some endocrine glands all work together to make up the immune system.

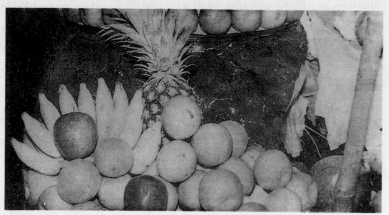
All kinds of fruits can greatly strengthen immune system.

A well functioning immune system is of great importance in the maintenance of good health. It can save a person from many health problems ranging from minor infections to cancer. The genetic makeup of a person greatly influences immune system. Environmental factors also exercise a lot of influence on it.

Diet is the most important factor in building up immunity. Foods contain vitamins, minerals and other important elements that can broadly stimulate immune functioning. This, in turn, will increase body resistance to various viral and bacterial infections, as well as cancerous growths that flourish or die according to the operation of immune mechanism.

FOODS THAT BUILD UP BODY RESISTANCE
Carrot, Curd or Yoghurt, Fruits & Vegetables, Garlic, Low-Fat Foods, Mushroom and Zinc-Rich Foods.

Carrot

A Carrot, as one of the richest sources of antioxidant beta-carotene, is a powerful immunity stimulating food. It strengthens immune defences against both bacterial and viral infections, as well as cancer. In one study of 60 older men and women, average age 56, beta-carotene increased the percentage of specific infection-fighting immune cells, such as natural killer cells and activated lymphocytes and T-helper cells. This study was conducted by Dr. Ronald R. Watson, Ph.D., at the University of Arizona in Tucson. It showed the more beta-carotene, the greater the increase in protective immune cells. For instance, both 30mg and 60mg of daily beta-carotene for two months improved immune cells, but the bigger dose was more powerful. Two months after the beta-carotene was stopped, the immune cells came down to pre-experiment levels. Such doses are comparable to eating five to ten carrots a day. Thus, a diet high in carotene-rich foods, such as carrots, could provide these immune-stimulating doses of beta-carotene. Other foods rich in carotene, besides carrot, are mangoes, papaya, orange, melon, green leafy vegetables, pumpkin, whole milk, curds and butter.

Curd or Yoghurt

Curd or Yoghurt is an extremely valuable immunity stimulating food. It has been regarded as an age-old fighter of disease and a powerful protector against viruses, infections and tumour cells. Eating curd stimulates at least two vital components of immunity, namely nature killer cells and gamma interferon. Dr. Joseph Scimeca, Ph.D., nutrition researcher at Kraft General Food Inc., explains that natural killer cells circulating in the body detect tumour cells, then seek out and destroy. Nature killer cells are one of the best defences against tumour cells and viruses, he says. Even Yoghurt that has been heated to kill 95 per cent of the bacterial cultures still activates nature killer cells, this was discovered by Dr. Scimeca.

A Remarkable proof in in this respect in human beings comes from research by Dr.Georges M. Halpern, M.D, of the University of California School of Medicine at Davis. In the first large-scale study of effects of yoghurt on immune system, Dr. Halpern and Colleagues found that those eating 450gm of yoghurt a day for four months had five times more infection-fighting gamma interferon in their blood than non-yoghurt eaters. In this study of 68 persons, age 20-40, one-third got no yoghurt, one-third got yoghurt with active live cultures and the remaining one-third got yoghurt that had been heated to destroy the live cultures. Only the yoghurt with live active cultures of lactobacillus bulgaricus and streptococcus thermophilus (standard in yoghurt worldwide) stimulated interferon.

If a person starts eating curd or yoghurt three months before pollen season or cold season, it can build up his immunity, considerably reducing his susceptibility to both these aggravations, says immunologist Dr. Halpern. In a year-long study of 120 young and elderly adults, he found that eating 170 grams of yoghurt a day significantly reduced the number of days the subjects had hay fever attacks, especially from grass pollens. The yoghurt eaters also had very few symptoms of hay fever and allergies. Further, those eating yoghurt daily had about 25 per cent less cold during a year than the non-yoghurt eaters.

Fruits & Vegetables

All kinds of fruits and vegetables can greatly strengthen immune system. Such plant foods contain a large number of compounds that can boost immunity, including vitamin C and beta-carotene. Vegetarians have more powerful immune defences. A recent study at the German Cancer Research Center in Heidelberg compared the blood of male vegetarians and meat eaters. They found that white cells of vegetarians were twice as deadly against tumour cells as those of meat eaters. This means vegetarians needed only half as many white cells to do the same job as meat eaters did. Researchers thought that vegetarian's white cells were more deadly, presumably due to their yielding greater armies of natural killer cells or more ferocious natural killer cells. Vegetarian also have higher levels of carotene in their blood, which greatly helps strengthen immune system.

Garlic

Garlic greatly helps stimulate immune functioning. Its anti-bacterial, antiviral and anti-cancer properties are partly

partly due to its ability to enhance immune functioning. It particu-larly stimulates the power of T-lymphocytes and macro-phages, which play a dominant role in immune functions. This has been discovered by Benjamin H.S. Lau, M.D., of the School of Medicine at Loma Linda University. In laboratory tests, he found that garlic extract impeled macrophages to generate more agents to kill microbes and tumour cells. Dr. Lau calls garlic a biological response modifier.

Several years ago, Dr. Tariq Abdullah, M.D., and colleagues at the Akbar Clinic and Research Center in Panama City, Florida, ate large amounts of raw garlic, up to 15 cloves a day. Others in the study ate no garlic. The blood from the garlic eaters had more natural killer cells. In fact, such natural killer cells, destroyed from 140-160 per cent more cells than did natural killer cells derived from non-garlic eaters. An amount as small as 1.8 grams of garlic, about half a clove, results in an increase in natural killer cell activity.

Low-Fat Foods

Too much fat, especially of the wrong type, weakens immune system. There is evidence to suggest that excessive fat impairs natural killer cell activity. One study at the University of Massachuetts Medical School by James R. Hebert, Sc.D., Associate Professor of Medicine and Epidemiology, had some young men decrease the fat in their diets on an average from about 32 per cent of calories to 23 per cent. Their natural killer activity increased about 48 per cent. Those who consumed the highest fat diets got the greatest immune boost from the reduction.

The vitality of the immune system also depends on the type of fat. Fish oil, containing omega-3 fatty acids, actually seems to strengthen immune system. Most harmful are the vegetable polyunsaturated fats called omega-6 fatty acids contained in corn, safflower and sunflower seed oils. Eating too much of them can severely disrupt immune functioning. For instance, such oils can inhibit formation of lymphocytes, causing a partial shutdown in immune responses.

Mushroom

Practitioners of traditional Chinese medicine have long hailed the healing power of the shiitake, the big, brown Asian mushrooms. In 1960, Dr. Kenneth Cochran, at the University of Michigan, discovered one reason for this. He isolated from the shiitake, antiviral susbstance called lentinin that showed a strong immunity-boosting activity.

Recent research by scientists at Semmelweis Medical University in Budapest, Hungary, have also found that lentinin can modify cells to resist the colonisation or spreading of lung cancer cells. Thus the shiitake mushrooms may help the immune system fight and prevent cancer.

Zinc-Rich Foods

Zinc-rich foods can enhance immunity functioning. This mineral helps increase many aspects of immunity, including production of antibodies and T-cells, as well as other white-blood-cell activity. It has been shown in experiments on animals that when they are deficient in zinc, they cannot fight off attacks by bacteria, viruses and parasites. It has also been observed that adults and children deficient in zinc, often have more colds and respiratory tract infections. According to Dr. Novera H. Spector, a scientist at the American National Institute of Health, zinc may even rejuvenate an ageing immune system. He explains that zinc may help reverse declining immune functions that dectiorate rapidly after the age of 60 years. After the middle age, the thymus gland, which plays a key role in immune defences, begins to decline radically. The thymus gland secretes thymulin, a hormone that stimulates production of T-cells. With the decline of thymus gland, the output of thymulin also decreases.

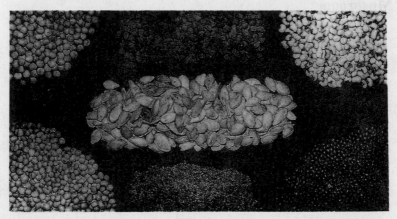

Zinc-rich foods like seeds can enhance immunity functioning.

Italian studies have discovered that even low doses of zinc, taken daily, resulted in an amazing 80 per cent regrowth of their thymus glands, a significant increase in active hormones and T-cells that fight infections. Dr. Nicola Fabris, Ph.D., at the Italian National Research Centre on Ageing in Ancona, gave 15mg of zinc daily to a small group of people over age 65. Their blood levels of hormones and active T-celis increased so high as to be equal to levels seen in young people. The main vegetarian food sources of zinc are milk, beans, whole grain cereals, nuts and seeds, especially pumpkin seeds.

CHAPTER 16

LIFE-PROLONGING FOODS

According to Dr. Edward Henderson, a past president of the American Geriatric Society, the age of one hundred is a realistic and conceivable goal. Dr. Thomas S.Gardiner, one of the founders of the National Foundation for Anti-ageing Research, believes that we have not even approached the normal span of life. He claims that most ageing is premature, and that body organs are designed to last six to seven times as long as it usually takes the average person to reach maturity. He believes that we could double the life span.

There are three most important factors, which determine the condition of our bodies and often the lengths of our lives. These are nutrition, activity and mental outlook. Nutrition is the most important factor contributing to good health and longevity. It is the basis of any programme designed to help a person stay young longer. The entire body from heart to brain, from cells and tissues to bloodstream, depends for their survival upon the food we eat.

FOODS THAT PROMOTE LONGEVITY

Alfalfa, Almond, Apple, Barley, Brahmi, Chebulic Myroblan, Curd or Yogurt, Garlic, Ginseng, Honey, Indian Gooseberry, Lettuce, Milk, Olive Oil, Onion, Pollen, Raw Foods, Rice (brown), Sage and Soyabean.

Alfalfa

Alfalfa, one of the most nutritionally versatile foods, is a valuable source of several vitamins and other food ingredients. It is a rich source of vitamin A, B, D, E and G. It also has some vitamin C and K.

Investigations made by the U.S. Department of Agriculture in recent years have revealed that alfalfa contains one and half times more protein than grains like wheat and corn and that its carbohydrate content is only half of that found in grains. The alfalfa proteins contain such essential amino acids as arginine, lysine, theronine and tryptophane. These amino acids are of paramount importance in maintaining good health and preventing deficiencies.

Of special value in alfalfa is the rich quality, quantity and proper balance of calcium, magnesium, phosphorus, chlorine, sodium, potassium and silicon. These elements are all very much needed for the proper functioning of the various organs in the body. This herbal food is one of the richest chlorophyll foods that build up both animals and humans into a healthy and vigorous old age. Its regular use can thus promote health and longevity.

This can be used either in the form of sprouted seeds, or in the form of juice extracted from the leaves or as herbal tea, made from the seeds as well as from dried leaves of the plant.

Almond

Almonds help built up both physical and mental health and prolong life. It is rich in all essential elements needed by the body. The medicinal virtues of almonds arise chiefly from pharmacodynamic action of copper, iron, phosphorus and vitamin B_1. These chemicals exert a synergetic action and help the formation of new blood cells, hemoglobin and plays a major role in maintaining the smooth physiological functions of brain, nerves, bones, heart and liver. Almonds are thus beneficial in preserving the vitality of the brain, in strengthening the muscles and in prolonging life. They form a vital part of all tonic preparations in Ayurveda and Unani Medicines.

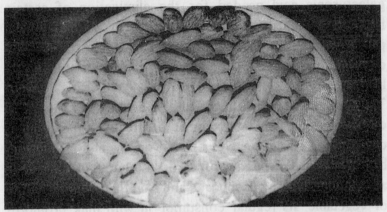

Almonds help built up both physical and mental health and prolong life.

The best way to use almonds is to soak them in water for few hours and grind them into fine paste after removing the skin. This paste is called almond butter. It is easily assimilated and is preferred to dairy butter by many vegetarians. This butter is of special value to older people who are generally bothered with the problem of not getting enough protein in their diets. By taking almond butter, they will be able to get not only high quality protein but also other excellent food ingredients, contained in the almond, in the most easily digestible form.

Apple
This popular fruit is a disease fighting food and helps

prolong life. It reduces cholesterol and helps prevent cancer. It possesses mild antibacterial, antiviral, anti-inflammatory and oestrogenic properties. This fruit is high in fiber and thus prevents constipation.

The active medicinal principle of apple is pectin, a natural therapeutic ingredient found in the inner portion of the rind and the pulp. Pectin aids in detoxification by supplying the galacturonic acid needed for the elimination of certain harmful substances. It also helps prevent putrefaction of protein matter in the alimentary canal. The malic acid contained in the apple is beneficial to the bowels, liver and brain.

The apple is the best fruit to tone up a weak and run-down condition of the human system. It is gifted with the qualities of removing all deficiencies of vital organs and making the body stout and strong. It tones up the body and the brain as it contains more phosphorus and iron than any other fruit or vegetable. Its regular consumption with milk promotes health and youthfulness and prolongs life.

Barley

Pearled barley has always been used by Oriental folk physicians for the healing and the rejuvenation of the digestive system. A simple, yet effective folk remedy was to make barley brew that could be sipped throughout the day while other foods were restricted or limited. This folk remedy has helped many people, even to this day.

To prepare this brew, one-quarter cup of all natural pearled barley should be boiled in two litres of water. It should be strained when half the water has evaporated. Drinking of this all-natural barley brew will relax the stomach. It helps digestive rejuvenation and benefits the digestive system in

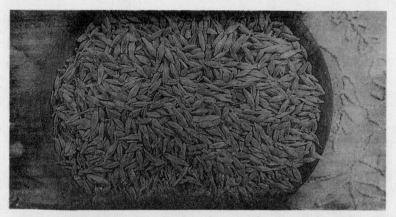

Pearled Barley helps healing and the rejuvenation of the diagestive system and thereby prolongs life.

two ways. It soothes the burning digestive actions and it introduces a natural oily substance, which helps protect the eroded mucous membrane of the digestive system. These benefits also help prevent the ageing process of the digestive system. Once the digestive system is thus soothed and healed, it can promote better assimilation of foods and thereby prolong life.

Brahmi

Brahmi, known as Indian pennywort, is a very popular Indian herb, with many medicinal virtues. It is a perennial wild creeper, which is prostate, small and smooth. It is very beneficial in correcting the disordered processes of nutrition and restoring the normal function of the system. All the parts of the creeper are used both for therapeutic and culinary purposes.

According to Pandit Devadutta Sharma of Asthang Ayurvedic College Culcutta, brahmi possesses the property of lengthening the life span much more than the effect it is known to have on increasing mental faculties like power of thinking and memory. It is said that a person named 'Jinchigiyan' of China attained the age of 250 years by the regular use of this Indian herb.

Many scientists abroad have been conducting researches on the ingredients and properties of brahmi for a long time. One eminent British scientist found that this small herb possesses the miraculous property of curing various diseases. He believes that for different diseases, it should be used in combination with different herbs, but if only its two leaves are taken daily, it adds to the vitality and longevity of man considerably.

The ancient medical book 'Vagbhatt' mentions that if a man fries little brahmi in ghee and takes it with milk regularly for a month and abstains from taking cereals, he can live for an exceptionally long period. Similarly the ancient medical treatise Charak Samhita mentions that if juice of brahmi is taken with one forth quantity of liquorice powder and milk, it cures all kinds of diseases and bestows longevity. The dosage varies according to the constitution of the user.

Chebulic Myroblan

Chebulic Myroblan is a miraculous herb and is known as long-life elixir. It has been used in Indian system of medicine for a very long time. The physicians in ancient India used it in the treatment of diarrhoea, dysentery, heartburn, flatulence, dyspepsia, liver and spleen disorders. There is an old Indian proverb, which says, 'If one bites a piece of *haritaki* everyday after meals and swallows its juice, he will remain free from all diseases.'

Chebulic myroblan is a mild, safe and efficacious laxative. It helps arrest secretion or bleeding and it strengthens the stomach and promotes its action. It is useful in correcting disordered processes of nutrition and restores the normal function of the system. This herb is thus highly valuable in maintaining good health and prolonging life.

Curd or Yogurt

Curd or yogurt is a lactic fermentation of milk. It is esteemed for its smoothness, its pleasant and refreshing taste. It is a highly versatile and health-promoting food and one of the most valuable therapeutic foods. Curd is a very nourishing food. It is a valuable source of protein, essential vitamins and minerals. It is also a rich source of calcium and riboflavin.

Curd has been associated with longevity. Prof. Elie Metchnikoff, a Noble prize-winning Russian bacteriologist at the Pasteur Institute, believed that premature old age and decay could be prevented by taking sufficient curd in the daily diet. He made an intensive study of the problem of old age in the early 1900s. He came to the conclusion that the body is slowly being poisoned and its resistance weakened by man's normal diet and that this poisoning process could be arrested and the intestinal tract kept healthy by the constant, regular use of yogurt or some variety of acidophilus milk.

Galen, one of the most famous of the Greek doctors, claimed that yoghurt was beneficial for a bilious and burning stomach and that it changed its nature by purifying it. He said that milk taken straight from the cow had heating and burning quality, but fermented milk did not. Yoghurt is far more easily digested than milk.

Dioscorides, another famous physician, commended the use of yoghurt as a medicament for the liver, stomach and blood tuberculosis as well as for infection of the nose, ears and uterus. Curd or yoghurt is thus, a food of great value in building of health and prolonging life.

Garlic

This important condiment crop has been held in high esteem for its health-building qualities for centuries all over the world. In herbal medicine, garlic has been traditionally used for numerous ailments. Babhet, an eminent Ayurvedic authority, is of the opinion that garlic is good for the heart, a food for the hair, a stimulant to appetite, a strengthening food, useful in leucoderma, leprosy, piles, worms, catarrhal disorders, asthma and cough.

Clinical experiments in recent times have confirmed several ancient ideas about healing value of this vegetable. These experiments have in fact shown much greater power of garlic than known previously. It lowers blood pressure, blood cholesterol, discourages blood clotting, fights cold and numerous other diseases, as well as helps prevent heart attacks. It contains multiple anti-cancer compounds and antioxidants. It also boosts immune system. Garlic is thus an all-round wonder drug, which builds up health, prevents and cures several ailments and prolongs life.

Ginseng

Ginseng is a wonder herb with outstanding medicinal properties. It has been used in China, Korea, Japan, India and Southeast Asia since ancient times for its health-building properties. It has been credited with vitalizing and restorative power, thereby prolonging life.

Orient folk physicians have asserted that a plant is effective against ailments of that organ, which shape it resemble. Of all their healing plants and herbs, ginseng is the only one that is shaped like a man. The people in the Orient believed that ginseng was a prime source of all the elements that would help rebuild a man's health and his powers of virility. Modern scientific studies on this herb found that it emits a mitogenetic ray, which is considered as an all-natural ultraviolet radiation. Nature has put within ginseng a process of cellular proliferation via this mitogenetic emission. It is said that this all-natural cellular rejuvenation process stimulates the body's own sluggish process and thereby promotes healing, cellular regeneration and longevity.

Ginseng is available in the form of powder or capsules. The powder can be used as a tea or added to fruit and vegetable juices. However, the Chinese prefer to chew a portion of the root everyday.

Honey

Honey is one of the most splendid foods. It possesses unique nutritional and medicinal properties. It is an excellent source of heat and energy. Energy is generated mainly by the carbohydrate foods and honey is the most easily digested form of carbohydrate. It enters directly into the bloodstream because of its dextrin content and this provides almost instantaneous energy. Those with weak digestion especially benefit form its use.

Latest research indicates that the pollen in honey contains all 22 amino acids, 28 minerals, two enzymes, 14 fatty acids and 11 carbohydrates. It thus builds up health, Wards off several common aliments and prolongs life.

Indian Gooseberry

This fruit has been used as a valuable ingredient of

various medicines in India and the Middle East since time immemorial. Shusrut, the great Ayurvedic authority, considers it as the best of all acid fruits and most useful in maintaining health and fighting disease. It contributes greatly towards good health and longevity. It is said that the great ancient sage Muni Chyawan rejuvenated himself in his late 70's and regained his virility by the use of Indian gooseberry.

Indian gooseberry has revitalising effects. It contains an element, which is very valuable in preventing ageing and in maintaining strength in old age. It improves body resistance and protects against infection. It strengthens the heart, hair and different glands in the body. It thus contributes greatly towards health and longevity.

Lettuce

This popular salad plant is a live food with its rich vitamin and mineral content, especially the antiscorbutic vitamin C. It is rich in mineral salts with the alkaline elements greatly predominating. So it helps keep the blood clean, the mind alert and body in good health.

Lettuce contains several health-building qualities and many medicinal virtues. It is very good for brain, nervous system and lungs. The raw juice of lettuce is cool and refreshing. The high content of magnesium in the juice has exceptional power to vitalise the muscular tissues, the nerves and the brain. This salad vegetable thus contributes greatly towards health and longevity.

Milk

Milk is one of the most common articles of food throughout the world. It occupies a unique position in the maintenance of health and healing of diseases. It is considered

as " Nature's most nearly perfect food."
Milk is regarded as a complete food. It contains protein,
fat, carbohydrates, all the known vitamins, various minerals
and all the food ingredients considered essential for sustaining
life and maintaining health. The protein of milk is of the
highest biological value and it contains all the amino acids
essential for body building and repair of body cells.
A litre of milk provides all the calcium needed by a person
for one day, practically all the phosphorus, a liberal amount
of vitamins A and C, one third or more of the protein, one
eight or more of the iron, at least one fourth of the energy,
and some of vitamins B, E and D. Milk ranks high in
digestibility. Its fat is 99 per cent digestible, its protein 97
per cent, and its carbohydrates 98 per cent. Milk is said to
require about one and half-hours for digestion.
According to Charaka, the great author of the Indian system
of medicine, milk increases strength, improves memory,
removes exhaustion, maintains strength and promotes long
life. Experiments conducted in modern times have amply
corroborated this opinion of Charaka.

Olive Oil

This mono unsaturated oil is regarded as a longevity
food. Its use is considered more beneficial for the heart
than low-fat diet, which is generally advocated by health
experts. Typically, the Mediterranean people eat more fat
than Americans, but about three-quarters of all their fat
come from monounsaturated fat, mostly from olive oil. They
also eat very little saturated animal fat. For example, residents
of the island of Crete sometimes drink olive oil by the glass,
deriving their quota of calories from fat to over 40 per cent.
Dr. Keys, professor at the University of Minnesota, found

in his remarkable "Seven Countries Study", that Cretans rarely succumbed to heart disease. In a 15-year period only 38 out of 10000 Cretans died of heart disease compared with 773 Americans, giving the United States 20 times as much deadly heart disease as Crete. Other Mediterranean populations also had low rates.

It has been observed that those Mediterranean people who consume olive-oil-type fat liberally were least to die of cancer or any other disease. Using mono unsaturated fat, as the major source of fat was the only dietary factor, according to Dr. Keys, that warded off death from all causes. It can thus be said that a relatively high-fat diet does not seem hazardous to the heart if it is very low in animal fat and high in olive-oil-type fat. Olive oil thus helps build up health and prolongs life.

Onion

Onion has been described by some one as the dynamite of natural foods. Compared with other fresh vegetables, it is relatively high in food value, moderate in protein content and is rich in calcium and riboflavin. It is considered as one of civilizations oldest medicines, which the ancient Mesopotamians believed as a cure for virtually every health problem. Onion is a powerful antioxidant food and contains numerous anticancer compounds. It thins the blood, lowers blood cholesterol, raises good-type HDL cholesterol, wards off blood clots, fights asthma, chronic bronchitis, hay fever, diabetes, atherosclerosis and infections. It also increases libido and strengthens the reproductory organs. This vegetable thus helps in maintaining good health and in preventing and curing several serious diseases, thereby prolonging life.

Pollen

Pollen is a fine powder, usually yellow in colour, found inside the blossoms of herbs and flowers. It has been mentioned in texts of Babylon, Egypt, Persia and China that this outstanding plant substance was highly beneficial in giving strength to the body, in maintaining good health and in prolonging life. Even today, several primitive tribes who live a more natural life, use it as a valuable remedy for several ailments and for staying young.

In 1945, Nicolai Titsin, a Russian Biologist, questioned 50 people in Russia who claimed to be over 100 years of age. He discovered that a large number of them were bee keepers and all of them ate waste matter in the bottom of the beehive, a large part of which was almost pure pollen.

Scientists in different countries have carried out experiments with pollen. They agree that hardly a foodstuff exists in either the vegetable or animal kingdom in which so many varied essentials of digestive needs are so completely united as in the case of pollen. Researchers in Switzerland have shown that it contains protein, free amino acids, various forms of sugar, mucilage, fats, minerals, trace elements, large amounts of of the vitamin B Complex and also vitamins A, D, E and C. It also contains numerous diastase, hormone components and antibiotics, besides other active ingredients not yet specified. They conclude that various elements contained in pollen work together to keep a person more youthful even in old age.

Raw Foods

Raw foods promote health and longevity. Before the discovery of fire, man's evolution and development depended on the consumption of natural, raw foods, as provided by nature. After fire came into existence, man started cooking natural foods without much thought. Cooking of natural foods led to their debasement and destruction of most of their essential nutrients needed for the maintenance of good health.

The nutritive constituents of raw foods serve as building material for the construction and renewal of cells. They produce energy to put these cells into motion and give warmth to the body and supply the raw materials to the specialised cells needed for their productive activities.

Those who eat raw foods make use of the digestive organs at about one-fourth of their potential capacity. As a result, their organs are never overloaded or fatigued. Because of the large quantities of mineral salts they contain, in a form most suitable to the needs of the system, fresh fruits and raw vegetables are known as purifying foods. They possess eliminating, cleansing and healing properties.

The adoption of raw eating can thus free mankind from all diseases. Raw foods contain all the essential vitamins, minerals, trace elements and other constituents, which help maintain good health, prevent disease and prolong life.

Rice (brown)

Brown rice has always been considered a marvelous healer in the East. In many ancient writings of the Orients, it is said that natural, whole-grain brown rice is a "perfect" healing food because it is so delicately balanced by Nature. Many ancient physicians of India believed that abstaining from most foods and subsisting on brown rice for a few days would create a balanced condition, which would promote better health and longevity. Similar evidences of the importance of rice as a source of health have been found in the early literature of Thailand, Burma, Malaya and Indochina. The Orientals have always recognized that rice could promote a feeling of well being and youthful health.

The health benefits of brown rice, as described by the ancient folk physicians, have been confirmed by modern scientists. Eating brown rice helps create serenity and tranquility. It contains all the elements needed to help create better health. Rice protein, which comprises up to eight per cent of the grain, has eight of the essential amino acids, out of about eleven, in a delicate balance. A complete internal rejuvenation takes place, when rice protein is metabolized into health-building amino acids. These amino acids build flexible muscles, healthy skin and hair and clearer eyesight. They also nourish the heart and lungs, tendons and ligaments, brain, nervous system and glandular network.

Natural brown rice is a prime source of the healthy B-complex vitamins. In particular, rice offers thaimine, riboflavin and niacin, which are needed to promote youthful energy and to nourish the skin and blood vessels. An abundance of minerals in natural brown rice helps nourish the hormonal system, heal wounds, create a healthy heartbeat and regulate blood pressure. In particular, rice has a high amount of calcium, which soothes and relaxes the nervous system and helps relieve symptoms of hypertension. Further, iron contained in rice, enriches the bloodstream. Rice offers phosphorus and potassium to work with other nutrients and maintain internal water balance. Brown rice thus helps maintain good health, wards off diseases and prolongs life.

Sage

This important culinary herb possesses many health-building properties. The Chinese saying 'sage for old age' sums up its healthful qualities. It has a reputation to retard old age, restore energy and aid digestion.

Sage has centuries-old reputation as a sacred plant capable of exerting a beneficial influence on the brain, nerves, eyes and glands. Gerard, the famous herbalist, wrote that he found sage effective for "quickening the senses and memory, strengthening the sinews and resorting health to those suffering from palsies of moist cause, removing, shaking and trembling of limbs". This herbal food is thus of great value as a promoter of health and longevity.

Sage is generally used as a flavouring agent. Dried and powdered leaves can be mixed with cooked vegetables. Fresh sage leaves can be used in salads and sandwiches. The young leaves are pickled, and used for making tea.

Soyabean

The soyabean is esteemed for its high food value. It is a very valuable source of protein, vitamins, minerals and other food ingredients. Its protein is of high biological value and is considered 'complete', as it contains all the essential amino acids. It is the best of all-vegetable proteins and ranks in this respect with protein of milk, eggs and meat. But soyabean contains by far more protein than these articles. The soyabean contains many medicinal virtues. While most of the proteins are acid in their ash, soyabean is rich in alkaline-bearing salts and hence regarded as a corrective diet. The high quality protein contained in soyabean helps build vigour, vitality and a feeling of youthful health.

The Chinese who consume soyabeans liberally, believe that it makes the body plump, improves the complexion, stimulates the growth and removes constipation and many other physical ailments. Modern researches carried out in the laboratories in Europe and America has corroborated much of these claims. The Chinese and Japanese often enjoy youthful living well beyond the century mark because they consume a large amount of soyabean in their diet.

The soyabean is one of the richest known sources of lecithin which is considered an amazing youth element. With sufficient intake of lecithin, cholesterol cannot build up against the walls of the arteries and veins. Besides reducing the cholesterol level in the blood, there is mounting scientific evidence to suggest several other benefits from lecithin. It has been suggested that its intake in sufficient amounts can help rebuild those cells and organs, which need it. Lecithin helps maintain their health once they are repaired. It may mean that a deficiency of lecithin in the diet may be one of the causes of ageing and that its use may be beneficial in retarding the ageing process and prolonging life.

CHAPTER 17

MEMORY ENHANCING FOODS

According to Dr. William Kountz, director of Scientific Research of Gerontological Research Foundation, St. Louis Missouri, "Allowing oneself to slip mentally as well as physically is the primary cause of deterioration. Memory loss is not a sign of ageing, but a sign of increasing carelessness." His advice is to keep the mind going by constant activity and proper diet.

Investigations conducted in several laboratories show that brain does not necessarily corrode with age, so long as it is free of actual disease. Researches over the past several years have shown that the human brain can grow in a variety of ways in a surprising manner, even in advanced old age. Neuroscientist, Dr.Robert Terry, M.D., of the University of California, has shown that the brain cells called neurons, which are responsible for processing information, do not really die off with age, they merely shrink. Although these smaller neurons do not function as well as larger ones, Dr. Terry thinks they might be regrown or retrained to work normally.

It is essential that the body is supplied with adequate food substances, such as proteins, carbohydrates, minerals, vitamins and hormones for proper physical and mental development. Pioneering new research studies reveal that foods can help determine mental alertness, memory and concentration.

FOODS THAT SHARPEN MEMORY
Almond, Apple, Asafoetida, Brahmi, Cumin Seeds, Lemon Balm, Pepper, Phosphorus-Rich Fruits, Rosemary, Sage and Walnut.

Almond

This most important nut is a valuable food for increasing memory. It is especially beneficial in the treatment of loss of memory due to brain weakness. It contains unique properties to remove brain debility and to strengthen it. This nut preserves the vitality of the brain and cures various disorders of the nervous system.

Almonds should be immersed in water for about two hours and their upper red coating removed. They should then be made into a fine paste by rubbing them on a stone slab with sandalwood and taken mixed with butter or alone. The most useful preparation of almonds, however, is the almond milk. It can be easily prepared by grinding the blanched almonds to a smooth paste and adding cold boiled water to the consistency of the milk. With the addition of little honey, it makes a delicious and nutritious drink. One litre of milk may be obtained from 250 grams of almonds. Inhaling 10 to 15 drops of almond oil through the nose is also beneficial in the treatment of dullness of memory resulting from brain weakness.

Apple

Apple is a memory enhancing food and is beneficial in the treatment of dullness of memory. The various chemical substances contained in it help control the wear and tear of nerve cells. Apple is of special value as a brain food to enhance memory due to its richness in trace mineral boron.

According to recent experiments by research psychologist Dr. James Penland, Ph.D., at the U.S. Department of Agriculture's Grand Forks Human Nutrition Research Centre, this trace mineral appears to affect the electrical activity of the brain. Lake of boron can subdue mental alertness, says Dr. Penland.

He put 15 people over the age of 45 alternately on a low-boron and high-boron diet for about four months. When the subjects ate little boron, the electrical activity in their brains was more sluggish, indicating a decrease in mental activity. "Their brains produced more theta waves and fewer alpha waves, which happens when you become drowsy," he says. The lack of boron seemed to "downshift their brains." When they went on a high-boron regimen, 3mg a day, their brain wave activity increased, as detected by electroencephalograms. Two apples contained 1mg of brain-stimulating boron. Eating an apple with honey and milk is very beneficial in lack of memory and concentration.

Asafoetida

This popular resinous gum is said to help regenerate the brain and the nervous system and there by help increase memory. It also helps tone up sluggish organs to create a feeling of youthful vitality. It can be used as a 'mind tonic' in the powdered form. One and half teaspoon of this powder should be dissolved in two cups of boiled water. It should be allowed to cool and then sipped several tablespoons while working. This gives a feeling of mental alertness and sharpens memory.

Brahmi

The leaves of the Brahmi, also known as Indian

pennyworts, are a remarkable food medicine for enhancing memory. They are believed to improve the receptive and retentive capacity of the mind. The powder of the leaves should be taken with milk in small doses for this purpose, as well as for mental weakness.

Another way to use Brahmi is to dry it in shade and grind in water, along with seven kernels of almond and four and half decigrams of pepper. It should then be strained and sweetened with honey. This mixture should be drunk every morning for a fortnight on an empty stomach to increase memory and concentration.

Cumin Seeds

This popular spice is a brain food. Its use has been found beneficial in the treatment of dullness of memory. Three grams of black cumin seeds should be mixed with 12 grams of pure honey and licked to enhance memory.

Lemon Balm

This important culinary herb is regarded as a memory enhancing food. It is said to be very valuable for brain and for strengthening the memory. It relieves brain fatigue, sharpens comprehension, lifts the heart from depression and raises the spirits. A cold infusion of the balm can be taken freely for this purpose. It is prepared by infusing about 30 grams of the herb in half a litre of cold water for 12 hours and then strained. It should be taken in small doses throughout the day. Lemon balm can also be used in the form of herbal tea made from its heart-shaped leaves.

Pepper

Pepper is one of the oldest and most important of all

spices. It is known as 'King of Spices'. It is stimulant, pungent, aromatic, digestive and nervine tonic. This is a valuable food for enhancing memory. A pinch of finely

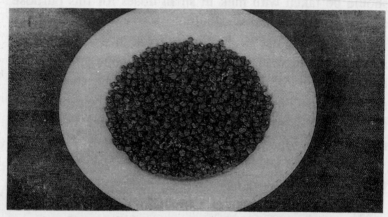

Pepper is a valuable food for enhancing memory.

ground pepper, mixed with honey, should be taken for this purpose. It should be taken both in the morning and evening.

Phosphorus-Rich Fruits
All the fruits, rich in phosphorus are valuable food to

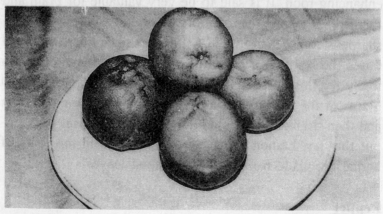

Phosphorous rich fruits like orange invigorate brain cells and tissues, thereby sharpen memory.

sharpen memory. Such fruits invigorate the brain cells and tissues. The fruits rich in this important mineral are figs, grapes, dates, orange, almond, walnut and apple. Their use is of special value in loss of memory due to brain weakness.

Rosemary

Rosemary is a sweet scented evergreen plant, which grows upto two meters high. It has long been regarded as the herb for the remembrance. It was once believed to strengthen the heart as well as the memory. The Greeks and Romans prepared a fragrant distilled water from the flowers and inhaled the odour so that "the evils were destroyed from the mind and the memory no longer played tricks." Dr. James a renowned physician wrote: "Rosemary is a plant of great service in affections of the head and nerves.... It strengthens the sight and memory."
Rosemary is considered as an antidote to mental fatigue and forgetfulness. In ancient Greece, students studying for their examinations threaded sprigs of rosemary in their locks to encourage clear thinking and a good memory. A tea made from the herb has been found highly beneficial for the businessmen and students who will find it refreshing and a good natural remedy for bringing added mental agility.
It is believed that if the crushed leaves of rosemary are inhaled, keeping the eyes closed, the mind will become crystal-clear as the plant's penetrating vapors seems to course through the brain cells.

Sage

This popular culinary herb is considered a useful remedy for failing memory. It has been found to have an action on cortex of the brain, which is said to be beneficial in mental exhaustion, strengthening the ability to concentrate. A tea made from the leaves should be taken to sharpen memory. This tea is prepared by pouring a cup of boiling water over dried sage leaves. The water should be covered and infused for several minutes. It should then be strained and sweetened with honey. In case of fresh leaves, a tablespoon of coarsely chopped sage leaves should be used and tea prepared in the same manner.

Walnut

Walnut is a unique dry fruit valuable in failing memory due to brain weakness. Its value will be enhanced if it is taken with figs or raisins. If it is intended to be consumed alone, about 20 grams of walnuts should be taken every day.

CHAPTER 18

MUCUS-CLEARING FOODS

It is been known for centuries that hot, spicy, pungent foods can help clear the lungs and breathing passages. They do so by thinning mucus and encouraging it to move along. When a person eats a hot food, his eye starts watering and his nose begins to run. The same thing happens in the lungs. It is considered that hot food activate nerve endings in the oesophagus and stomach, causing the watery reactions.

These age-old food remedies, passed down for centuries by medical practitioners and grandmothers, have stood the test of scientific investigations, especially inrespect of respiratory problems, like colds and flu. Dr. Irwin Ziment, M.D., professor of Medicine at UCLA has made comprehensive studies about these remedies. His study of early medical literature has lead him to conclude that foods used to fight respiratory diseases for centuries are very similar to the drugs being now used. They have a common action. They thin out and help move the lung's secretions so they do not congest air passages and can be coughed up or expelled in a normal way. Such foods and drugs are called "mucko-inetic", meaning mucus-moving agents, and include decongestants and expectorants. The most important of such foods for respiratory diseases are the chilli pepper and other hot and pungent foods. Even Hippocrates, the father of medicine prescribed vinegar and pepper to relieve respiratory infections.

FOODS THAT CONTROL RESPIRATORY DISEASES

Aniseed, Asafoetida, Bishop's Weed, Bitter Gourd Root, Chilli Pepper, Clove, Endive, Fennel, Figs (Dry), Garlic, Ginger, Holy Basil, Honey, Indian Gooseberry, Linseed, Mustard Seeds, Onion, Orange, Safflower Seeds, Sesame seeds, Spinach, Tamarind, Turmeric and Vitamin C-rich food.

Aniseed

This popular spice is a valuable mucus clearing food. It possesses expectorant property and helps remove phlegm from the bronchial tube. This property emanates from the essential oil contained in it. It can thus be beneficially used in respiratory system diseases like asthma, bronchitis and emphysema.

Aniseed is mostly used as a flavouring agent. It should not be boiled too long as it may lose its properties and essential oil during the process.

Asafoetida

Asafoetida possesses expectorant properties and it helps remove catarrhs and phlegm from the bronchial tube.

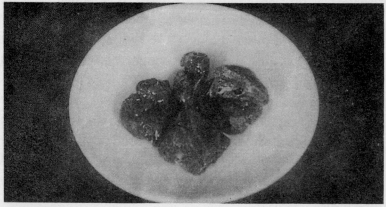

Asafoetida helps remove catarrhs and phlegm from the bronchial tube.

It thus helps control respiratory disorders like whooping cough, asthma and bronchitis. About 3 to 6 centigrams of this gum, mixed with 2 teaspoons of honey, a quarter teaspoon of white onion juice and 1 teaspoon of betel leaf juice, taken thrice daily will be highly beneficial in prevention and treatment of these disorders.

Bishop's Weed

This popular spice is a mucus clearing food and hence highly beneficial in the treatment of respiratory diseases. The seeds, mixed in buttermilk, make an effective medicine for relieving difficult expectoration caused by dried up phlegm. The seeds are also efficacious in bronchitis. A hot fomentation with the seeds is a popular household remedy for asthma. Chewing a pinch of *ajwain* seeds with a crystal of common salt and a clove is a very effective medicine for cough caused by acute pharyngitis in influenza.

Bitter Gourd Root

The roots of the bitter gourd plant possess mucus-clearing property. They have been used in folk medicine for asthma since ancient times. A teaspoon of the root paste, mixed with an equal amount of honey or juice of the holy basil, acts as an excellent expectorant medicine for this disease. It should be given once every night for a month.

Chilli Pepper

Hot chilli pepper is the best mucokinetic food among all hot spicy foods. According to Dr. Ziment, since antiquity, the flavoured foods for treating pulmonary and respiratory diseases have been mustard, garlic and hot chilli peppers. The active agents in these foods may work by several mechanisms. However, Dr. Ziment believes that they generally activate a flash flood of fluids in air passages that thin out mucus, so that it flows more easily.

As the hot stuff hits the mouth, throat and stomach, it touches nerve receptors that send messages to the brain, which in turn, stimulate the vagus nerve controlling secretion-producing glands that line the airways. The glands instantly release waves of fluids that can make the eyes water and the nose run. Dr. Ziment says that common pharmacological traits of all hot, pungent foods break up congestion, flushing out sinuses and washing away irritants. He prescribes hot foods for any condition in which secretions in the airways are thicker than normal, including sinusitis, a lump with congestion, asthma, hay fever, emphysema and chronic bronchitis.

Dr. Ziment also advises those who already suffer from chronic bronchitis and emphysema to eat hot food regularly, at least three times a week. He says that his patients who do so breathe more easily and require less treatment. Further, in surveys, he finds that those who eat more hot spicy cuisine are less likely to develop chronic bronchitis and emphysema, even if they smoke.

Dr. Ziment says, "A lot of drugs for colds and coughs and bronchitis do exactly what chilli peppers do, but I believe more in peppers. Peppers don't cause any side effects. I am convinced that 90 per cent of all people can tolerate hot food and get a benefit".

Clove

This popular herb possess mucus clearing property. It is thus an effective remedy for asthma and bronchitis. A teaspoon of decoction prepared by boiling 6 cloves in 30 ml of water makes an excellent expectorant medicine. It should be taken with honey three times daily for treating this condition.

Cloves are used as a table spice. They are mixed with other spices in the preparation of curry powder. They are also used to flavour the betel quid *(paan)*.

Endive

The juice of this vegetable is a valuable food for clearing mucus. Its use has been found especially beneficial in the treatment of asthma and hay fever. For better results, this juice should be combined with the juices of celery and carrot. This will serve as an excellent medicine, provided milk and foods containing concentrated starches and sugars such as white rice, white flours, macaroni, sweets, pastries and cakes are eliminated from the diet. The powder of the dry root is a very useful expectorant in chronic bronchitis. It should be given in doses of half a teaspoon, mixed with honey, thrice daily.

Fennel

The leaves and seeds of fennel possess mucus clearing properties. They promote the removal of catarrhal matter and phlegm from the bronchial tubes. They are thus beneficial in the treatment of respiratory disorders like asthma and bronchitis. The juice of the leaves may be given for treating these diseases. Eating fennel seeds with figs is also a good medicine for cough, bronchitis and lung abscesses.

Figs (Dry)

Dry figs help clear mucus from bronchial tube and are therefore a valuable food remedy for asthma. Phlegmatic cases of cough and asthma can be treated with success by their use. It gives comfort to the patient by draining off the phlegm. Three or four dry figs should be cleaned thoroughly with warm water and soaked overnight. They should be taken first thing in the morning, along with the water in which they are soaked. This treatment may be continued for about two months.

Garlic

Garlic is an excellent mucus clearing food. It is an effective expectorant and helps remove mucus from the bronchial tube. Allicin, which gives garlic its flavour, is converted in the body to a drug similar to S-carboxymethylcysteine (mucodyne), a classic European lung medication that regulates mucus flow.

Egyptians and Romans in ancient times and Arabs and Persians in medieval times, all used garlic to treat asthma. Even conventional physicians in Germany and United States used it as a remedy for asthma in the first half of the twentieth century. The biochemical mechanism involved may be that garlic affects substances called prostaglandins in the body. To derive this benefit, garlic must be heated or cooked. An effective method to take garlic in asthma is to boil three cloves in 30 ml. of milk and take once daily. Steaming ginger tea with minced garlic cloves in it can also help keep the problem under control and should be taken both in the morning and evening.

For a catarrh, garlic works wonder. Raw garlic will clear even the most intolerant choking mucus within a few hours only. It appears to do this by drying up the secretions and by killing the infections that are causing the mucus.

Ginger

Ginger is an expectorant food. It helps clear phlegm from the bronchial tube and is thus valuable in asthma, bronchitis and tuberculosis of the lungs. A teaspoon of fresh ginger juice, mixed with a cup of fenugreek decoction and honey to taste, is an excellent medicine in treatment of these conditions. The decoction of fenugreek is prepared by mixing one tablespoon of fenugreek seeds in a cupful of water. This mixture of ginger juice and fenugreek decoction should be taken both in the morning and evening.
A specific remedy for treating bronchitis is a mixture of half a teaspoon each of the powder of ginger, pepper and cloves. This mixture should be taken thrice daily. It may be licked with honey or taken as an infusion.

Holy Basil

The leaves of holy basil possess expectorant properties. They help remove catarrhal matter and phlegm from the bronchial tubes. They are thus useful in respiratory system disorders. Their decoction, with honey and ginger is an effective remedy for bronchitis, asthma, influenza, cough and cold. A decoction of the leaves, cloves and common salt also gives immediate relief in case of influenza. They should be boiled in half a litre of water till only half the water is left.

Honey

Honey is a mucus clearing food. It helps remove mucus and phlegm form bronchial tube. It is said that if a jug of honey is held under the nose of asthma patient and he inhales the air that comes into contact with honey, he starts breathing easier and deeper. The effect lasts for about an hour or so.

Honey usually brings relief whether the air flowing over it is inhaled or whether it is eaten or taken either in milk or water. It thins out accumulated mucus and helps its elimination from the respiratory passages. It also prevents the production of further mucus.

Indian Gooseberry

Indian Gooseberry is of great value as a mucus clearing food. It has proved beneficial in the treatment of respiratory systems disorders like asthma, bronchitis and tuberculosis of the lungs. Five grams of gooseberry juice, mixed with one tablespoon of honey, forms an effective medicinal expectorant tonic for the treatment of these diseases. It should be taken every morning. When fresh fruit is not available, dry gooseberry powder can be taken with honey.

Linseed

Linseed is a mucus clearing food. A decoction made from it is considered useful in curing congestion in asthma and prevent recurrence of attacks. This decoction is prepared by boiling a teaspoon of linseed powder and a piece of palm candy in two cups of water till the mixture is reduced to half. This decoction taken with a tablespoon of milk will give relief from chest congestion. Simultaneously linseed poultice should be applied externally at the lung bases for reducing internal congestion.

Mustard Seeds

Mustard seeds have been recognized for centuries as a decongestant and an expectorant. They help break up mucus in air passages. They are thus an effective remedy for congestion caused by colds and sinus problems. One

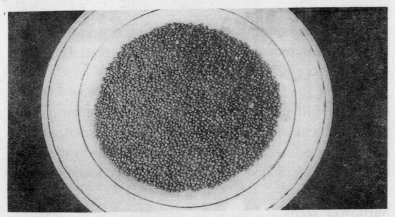

Mustard seeds have been recognised for centuries as a decongestant and an expectorant.

reason why mustard seeds are mucus clearing food is that it constitute a hot food.

During an attack of asthma and bronchitis, mustard seed oil, mixed with little camphor, should be massaged over the back of the chest. This will loosen up phelgm and ease breathing. The patient should also inhale steam from the boiling water mixed with caraway seeds. It will dilate the bronchial passage.

Onion

This popular vegetable is of great value as a mucus clearing food. It liquefies phlegm and prevents its further formation. It has been used as a food remedy for centuries in cold, cough, bronchitis and influenza. Equal amounts of onion juice and honey should be mixed together and three to four teaspoons of this mixture should be taken daily in treating these conditions. It is one of the safest preventive medicines against common cold during winter.

Orange

The juice of orange is an effective expectorant food. It helps clear mucus from the bronchial tube. This juice, mixed with a pinch of salt and a tablespoon of honey, forms an effective food medicine for respiratory systems disorders like tuberculosis of the lungs, asthma, common cold, bronchitis and other conditions of cough associated with difficult expectoration. Due to its saline action in the lungs, it eases expectoration and protects from secondary infection.

Safflower seeds

Safflower seeds possess mucus clearing property. They are especially beneficial in the treatment of bronchial asthma. Half a teaspoon of the powder of dry seeds, mixed with a tablespoon of honey, can be taken once or twice with great benefit in treating this disease. It acts as an expectorant and reduces the spasms by liquefying the tenacious sputum. An infusion of the flowers, mixed with honey, is also useful in asthma.

Sesame Seeds

Sesame seeds are an expectorant food. Their use have been found beneficial in the treatment of respiratory systems' disorders, especially acute and chronic bronchitis, asthma and pneumonia. An infusion of the seeds can be made by steeping 15 g of seeds in 250 ml of water. This infusion, mixed with a tablespoon of linseed, a pinch of common salt and a dessertspoon of honey, makes an excellent medicine for treating these diseases. This will help remove catarrhal matter and phlegm from the bronchial tubes.

Spinach

This popular green leafy vegetable possesses mucus clearing property and helps control respiratory diseases. An infusion of fresh leaves of spinach prepared with two teaspoon of fenugreek seeds, mixed with a pinch of ammonium chloride and honey, is an effective expectorant tonic. It can be given with beneficial results in the treatment of bronchitis, tuberculosis of the lungs, asthma and dry cough due to congestion in the throat. It soothes the bronchioles, liquefies the tenacious sputum and forms healthy tissues in the lungs and increases resistance against respiratory infections. It should be taken in doses of 30 ml. three times daily.

Tamarind

Tamarind-pepper 'rasam' is considered a food of exceptional value in clearing mucus. It is used as an effective home remedy for cold in South India. It is prepared by boiling for a few minutes, very dilute tamarind water in a teaspoon of hot ghee and half a teaspoon of black pepper powder. This steaming hot 'rasam' has a flushing effect. As one takes it, the nose starts running and eyes begin to water. This enables the nasal passage to become clear.

Turmeric

Turmeric is a valuable expectorant food. It helps clear mucus from the bronchial tubes. It is thus an effective food medicine in bronchial asthma. The patient should be given a teaspoon of turmeric powder mixed in a glass of milk, two or three times daily. It acts best when taken on an empty stomach.

Vitamin C-rich Foods

Vitamin C-rich foods are considered very valuable in clearing mucus. They help control respiratory diseases. A recent major study on 9000 adults by Dr. Schwartz supports this view. He discovered that people who ate foods containing 300mg of vitamin C a day were only 70 per cent as likely to have chronic bronchitis or asthma as those eating foods with one-third that much, or about 100mg. The difference is found in 225ml of orange juice. Foods rich in vitamin C are citrus fruits, green leafy vegetables, Indian gooseberry, sprouted Bengal grams and green grams.

CHAPTER 19

OESTROGENIC FOODS

Numerous plants contain phytoestrogens that are similar in molecular structure to that of human oestrogen. They have, however, a weaker and different effect. Plant oestrogen, being thus less powerful, is comparatively slow in generating benefits. But they are safer than synthetic oestrogen, which may produce adverse side effects. Moreover, some foods, notably vegetables of the cabbage family, increase the rate at which body burns up and disposes off oestrogen circulating in the body. Legumes, especially soyabeans, have particularly strong oestrogenic activity, and are now the commercial source for compounds used to make birth control pills.

Research studies show that there are at least 300 plants, many of them edible, which possess "Oestrogenic Activity". They help regulate the female hormone oestrogen.

FOOD THAT REGULATE HORMONE OESTROGEN

Beans, Cabbage, Low-fat Foods, Peanuts, Soyabean and Wheat bran.

Beans

Beans possess oestrogenic activity. Their consumption may help protect women from breast cancer. This is presumably due to the fact that they contain so-called phytoestrogens that help block the activity of cancer-promoting oestrogen. This opinion has been expressed by researcher Dr.Leonard A. Cohen, Ph.D., at the American Health Foundation in Newyork. Dr. Cohen says that Hispanic women in the Caribbean and Mexico are known to have less breast cancer than American women. In a new study, Dr. Cohen believes he has found the reason for this. According to him, Hispanic women eat twice as many beans, as American women.

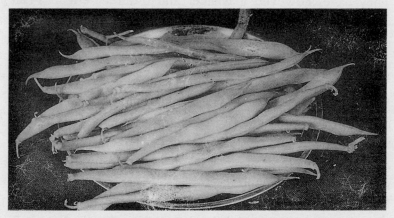

Beans possess oestrogenic activity and their consumption may help protect women from breast cancer.

Hispanic women consume over 115 grams of beans daily for six days a week, compared with same quantity of beans consumed by African-American women three times a week and twice a week for white American Women. Beans also possess several anti-cancer compounds, including protease inhibitors and phytates, say Dr. Cohen.

Cabbage

Cabbage and other cruciferous vegetables possess oestrogenic activities. They manage oestrogen and thereby help immunise against breast cancer. These vegetables can hasten the removal of oestrogen from the body, by speeding up its metabolism and burning up the hormone, so that less is available to feed cancer. This has been fully explained in chapter 11 on cancer fighting foods.

Low Fat Food

The amount of fats eaten in the diet also helps regulate both female and male hormones. A fatty diet may play havoc with a man's hormones and thus, his sex life. The quantity of fat women eats also influences oestrogen levels. A high-fat diet increases oestrogen. Thus cutting back on fat seems to check breast cancers, and perhaps other hormone-dependent cancers, by giving them less oestrogen to feed on. Several studies show that both premenopausal and postmenopausal women who reduce fat significantly, say from 35-40 per cent of calories to 20 per cent, have a substancial drop in blood oestrogen levels.

Peanuts

Peanuts, as a rich source of mineral boron, possess

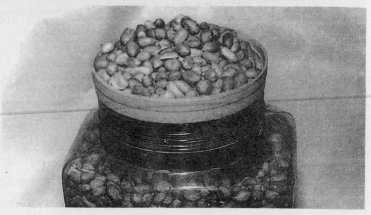

Peanuts, as a rich source of mineral boron, possess oestrogenic property.

oestrogenic property. Eating boron-rich food can boost oestrogen levels in postmenopausal women to a remarkable degree. The extent to which levels of oestrogen can be raised by taking such foods equals oestrogen replacement therapy. This has been reviled by a study conducted by U.S. Department of Agriculture researcher Dr. Forrest Nielson. According to him, boron seems to work, by increasing steroid hormones in the blood. He discovered that in women getting adequate amounts of boron, the most active form of oestrogen, oestradiol 17B doubled, reaching levels found in women on oestrogen replacement.

Soyabean

This vegetable is of great value as an oestrogenic food. It contains some compounds that can manipulate oestrogen. It can also directly inhibit the growth of cancerous cells, thereby reducing the risk of breast cancer in women. This has been explained in Chapter 11 on 'Cancer Fighting foods'.

Soyabeans offers a special type of lecithin, unlike lecithin found in other foods. Soyabean lecithin contains an abundance of auxines, identified as "vegetable hormones," which nourish and replenish the glandular system and help them pour forth youth-building hormones.

Wheat bran

Wheat bran possesses oestrogenic activity. It helps curtail oestrogen levels in blood and thereby reduce the risk of breast cancer. This however does not apply to other cereal brans like oat bran and corn bran. The main difference is that wheat bran fibre is highly insoluble, giving bacteria in the colon much to chew on. That, through an intricate series of biological events, causes less oestrogen to be released back into the bloodstream. Some authorities believe that the wheat bran would curb oestrogen, blocking cancer promotion in older, postmenopausal women also.

In fact, wheat fibre can suppress blood oestrogen even better than a low-fat diet does, according to a study at Tufts University School of Medicine. Investigator Margo Woods reported that both cutting fat and increasing fibre checked one type of oestrogen, namely oestrone sulphate, but only fibre reduced levels of oestradiol, which is considered to be a major villain in breast cancer. In animals, low fat, high-wheat fibre diet cuts the incidence of breast tumours to half. Other studies find that women who eat high-fibre diets have lower rates of breast cancer.

CHAPTER 20

PAIN KILLING FOODS

Certain foods can prevent perception of pain. This has been disclosed by recent researches on two common food compounds that can obstruct the perception of pain. One of these food compounds is caffeine. It has been recently discovered to be a mild painkiller, besides its common use in combination with other analgesic drugs. The other food compound is capsaicin, the hot chemical in chilli peppers. This is now being widely tested as a potential painkiller. For years people have put hot pepper extract on their gums to alleviate toothache. Now it is known that capsaicin in peppers serves as a local anesthetic and a promising new painkiller. Capsaicin suppresses pain by draining nerve cells of something called substance P, which relays pain sensations to the central nervous system. Thus, capsaicin helps block the perception of pain. Recently, the hot pepper essence has been injected or made into medications to help several diseases characterised by pain.

FOODS THAT RELIEVE PAIN

Asafoetida, Bishop's Weed, Clove, Ginger, Liquorice, Margosa, Mustard Seeds, Nutmeg, Onion and Poppy Seeds.

Asafoetida

This popular spice is a painkilling food. It is especially useful in relieving toothache. Asafoetida should be pestled in lemon juice and slightly heated. A cotton piece, soaked in this lotion should be placed in the cavity of the affected tooth. It will relieve pain quickly.

Bishop's Weed

Bishop's weed possesses pain-killing property. It is especially beneficial in treating earache. About half a teaspoon of the seeds should be heated in 30 ml of milk till the essence of the seeds permeate the milk. The milk is then filtered and used as ear drops. It decreases congestion and relieves pain.

The oil extracted from the seeds is an effective remedy for treatment of rheumatic and neuralgic pains. It should be applied on the affected parts.

Clove

This popular spice is a valuable painkilling food. It can be used beneficially in relieving pain in case of toothache. It helps decrease infection due to its antiseptic property. Clove oil, applied to a cavity in a decayed tooth, also relieves toothache. A clove sauted in a teaspoon of sesame oil and 3 to 5 drops of this warm oil put into the ear can cure earache. Muscular cramps are often relieved when the oil of clove is applied as a poultice on the affected part.

A paste of clove and salt crystals in milk is a common household remedy for headaches. Salt, as a hygroscopic agent, absorbs fluid and decreases tension.

Ginger

Ginger is an excellent painkiller. It can cure all types of pain. In headache, an ointment made from ginger, by rubbing dry ginger with a little water affords relief. This ointment should be applied to the forehead. It relieves toothache when applied to the face. In case of earache, a few drops of ginger juice instilled in the affected ear will give relief.

Liquorice

This well-known spice possesses pain killing property. It has been found especially helpful in muscular pains. An infusion should be prepared by soaking the dry roots overnight in water. This infusion should be given to the patients suffering from muscular pains. It is also very useful in chronic joint problems. It serves as cortisone in treating these conditions.

Margosa

The leaves of this popular tree are a pain killing food. Steam fomentation with *neem* decoction provides immediate comfort in cases of earache. A handful of leaves should be boiled in a litre of water and the ear fomented with the steam thus produced. The juice of *neem* leaves, mixed with an equal quantity of pure honey, is an effective remedy for boils in the ear. The juice should be warmed a little and a few drops instilled in the ear. Regular application for a few days will provide relief.

Mustard Seeds

Mustard is a pain killing food and a rubefacient. Its plaster or paste made with water is applied as an analgesic in rheumatism, sciatica, paralysis of limbs and other muscular pains. The plaster should, however, never be directly applied to the skin as it may cause painful blistering. A layer of linen material should be put between the mustard paste and the skin.

Nutmeg

This spice is of great value as a pain killing food. A nutmeg coarsely powdered and fried in *til* oil until all the particles become brown, is very useful as an external application to relieve rheumatic pains, neuralgia and sciatica. The oil should be cooled and strained before application.

Onion

Onion possesses pain killing property. It is beneficial in the treatment of pain in eye. The juice of onion and honey should be mixed in equal quantity and stored in a bottle. This mixture should be applied to the eyes by means of an eye-rod. It will provide relief in a short time.

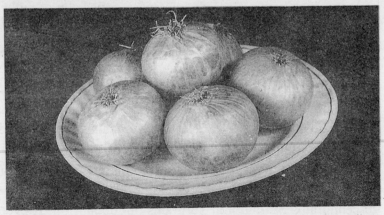

Onion is a valuable medicine for suppressing pain resulting from piles.

Onion is a valuable medicine for suppressing pain resulting

from piles. Occasionally, blind piles swell up and cause tortuous pain to the patient. It becomes extremely difficult for the patient even to sit. For treating this condition, two onions should be half-baked by burying them in live ash. They should then be thoroughly pounded into a paste after removing their outer covering. This paste should be fried in ghee and a tablet prepared from it. This tablet should be placed over the piles while hot. It should be retained there in position by applying a suitable dressing. The patient will feel comfort immediately after this application.

Poppy seeds

Poppy seeds on the stalks, which have not been slit to produce opium have sedative properties and are used for relieving pain. They can be used beneficially in griping pains after childbirth, colic and pain in the testicles.

Opium is useful in rheumatism, tumours of different kinds, cancers, carbuncles, abscesses, ulcers, leprosy, syphilis or scrofula, a disease characterised by tuberculosis of the lymph node in which pain causes sleeplessness, especially at night. The commencing dose is 6 centigrams of the extract. If it is insufficient, upto 18 centigrams may be advised to those who are unaccustomed to opium. Beyond this, it is unsafe to go without any professional advice. This may be combined with 12 or 18 centigrams of camphor. Opium is very effective in spasms of bowels. It is also useful in relieving pain and irritation of the bladder caused by stone.

Opium is useful as a liniment for soothing, both muscular and neuralgic pains. The liniment can be prepared by mixing 90 centigrams of opium in 15 grams of coconut oil. It even soothes painful piles. In painful teeth cavities, a centigram of opium is put into the hollow of the tooth. Care should, however, be taken not to swallow the saliva.

CHAPTER 21

SEX STIMULATING (APHRODISIAC) FOODS

The use of love potions to stimulate sexual power and stamina made from natural foods and other substances are as old as human race. The ancient Chinese healers even before 2000 B.C., were boiling the root of a plant known as jen shen and giving the brew to men whose sexual ambitions far exceeded their sexual capacities.

In ancient Babylon, women were munching candy made of sesame seed and honey for sexual health and fertility. For countless generations, the Hungarian gypsies and the mountain-dwelling Bulgarians have been eating pumpkin seeds to preserve the health of prostate gland and thereby male potency.

The modern researchers have established the efficacy of many of these natural remedies to correct sexual inadequacy and dysfunction. The natural foods and other substances described herein are the rich sources of nutrients needed for building the health of various sex glands and organs of the reproductive system.

FOODS THAT PROMOTE SEXUAL HEALTH

Almond, Asafoetida, Asparagus, Banyan, Bengal gram, Betel Morsel, Bishop's Weed, Black gram, Cardamom, Carrot, Cowhage, Dates (dried), Drumstick Flowers, Fenugreek Seeds, Garlic, Ginger, Ginseng, Honey, Indian Gooseberry, Jambul Fruit, Lady's Finger, Mango, Musk Melon, Nutmeg, Onion, Pepper (Black), Pumpkin Seeds, Raisins (Black), Safflower Seeds, Sesame Seeds and Wheat Germ Oil.

Almond

This most popular nut is very useful in case of loss of. sexual energy, which usually results from nervous debility and brain weakness. Its regular use will strengthen sexual power. It has the property to strengthen brain faculties and make the body stout and strong. Chewing of equal quantity of almond kernels and roasted Bengal gram also help in restoring sexual vigour.

Asafoetida

This popular resinous gum and flavouring agent, with pungent smell, is a powerful sex stimulating food. It is thus beneficial in the treatment of impotency. About 6 centigrams of asafoetida should be fried in ghee and mixed with honey and a teaspoon of fresh latex of banyan tree. This mixture makes a very effective sex tonic. It should be taken once daily for 40 days before sunrise in treating sexual debility and impotence. It is also considered a specific medicine for spermatorrhoea and premature ejaculation.

Asparagus

This vegetable is of great importance in the diet because of its valuable salts and vitamins as well as its large amount of cellulose contents. It is a highly alkaline food, with multipurpose therapeutic properties. It is considered a valuable aphrodisiac food. Known to have cultivated by the Greeks, it remained a favourite even with the Arabs for centuries together. Arabs believe that boiling it in water, then frying it in fat for a short time and sprinkling it with condiments makes a powerful sex stimulant.

One of the reasons why asparagus is considered aphrodisiac is because it is rich in iodine, and Iodine-rich foods do a lot to stimulate erotic energy. Iodine stimulates the endocrine glands, especially the thyroid. The thyroid glands produce thyroxin necessary for a good metabolism, good skin tone, and a good sex drive.

In India the dried roots of asparagus are used in Unani medicine as an aphrodisiac. It is available in the market as *safed musli*. About fifteen grams of the roots boiled in a cup of milk should be taken twice daily. Its regular use thickens the semen and is valuable in impotency and premature ejaculation.

Banyan

The banyan tree is a well-known popular tree grown all over India. It is used in traditional medicine for the treatment of several ailments. According to Ayurveda, the fruit of this tree is blood and semen producing food. This fruit can be obtained easily. It is more effective than many costly medicines in respect of its wonderful sex stimulating properties.

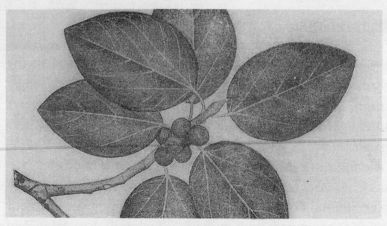

The fruit of the banyan tree is a blood and semen producing food.

The red and fully ripe fruits of the banyan tree should be collected from the branches. Those, which have fallen on the ground by themselves or have ever been in contact with iron, should never be used. These fruits should be spread on a piece of cloth in an airy shed to dry. They should then be rubbed into a fine powder with the help of a stone mortar or by hand manipulation and kept carefully after mixing with an equal quantity of sugar. This powder should be taken in doses of six grams with a little milk, both in the morning and evening. It makes the complexion rosy like the fruits themselves and is an unfailing remedy for premature ejaculation.

Tender roots of the Banyan tree are also considered beneficial in the treatment of female sterility. These roots should be dried in the shade and finely powdered. This powder should be mixed 5 times its weight with milk, and taken at night for 3 consecutive nights after menstruation cycle every month, till the conception takes place. No other food should be taken with this medicine.

Bengal Gram

Bengal gram also known as chicken Peas, is one of the most important pulses in India. It is consumed in the form of whole dried seeds and in the form of *dhal*. Bengal gram has many medicinal properties. Soaked in water overnight and chewed in the morning with honey, the whole gram seed acts as a general tonic.

The flour of the puffed Bengal gram is a very nutritive food and an effective remedy for impotency and premature ejaculation. For better results, two tablespoons of this flour should be mixed with honey, powdered dry dates and skimmed milk powder.

Betel morsel

Ayurvedic physicians prescribed betel morsel as an aphrodisiac food. Partly owing to its deodorant, aphrodisiac, and invigorating properties, *pan-supari* came to form a part of the ritual with which a wife welcomed her husband. The leaves are chewed together with betel nut as a masticatory. In its simplest form, sliced betel nut is wrapped in a betel leaf, smeared with lime (*Chuna*), katechu (*Katha)* and chewed. Often, a clove and other spices such as cinnamon and cardamom are also added. When chewed after meals, it sweetens the breath and acts as a gentle sex stimulant.

Bishop's Weed

Bishop's weed, one of the most popular spices, is credited with aphrodisiac properties. *Ajwain* seeds, combined with kernel of tamarind seeds, make a very effective sex tonic. Both these seeds in equal quantities should be fried in pure ghee, powdered and preserved in airtight containers. A teaspoon of this powder, mixed with a tablespoon of honey, should be taken daily with milk before retiring. It will increase virility and cures premature ejaculation. This remedy is far more effective than many costly medicines. Moreover, it enables the semen to impregnate the women by the production of sparmatoza in it. The use of this remedy will also bless the person with a healthy child.

Black gram

This popular pulse is considered as a sex stimulating food. It should be soaked in water for about six hours and then fried in pure cow's ghee, after draining the water. It makes an excellent sex tonic. It can be used with wheat bread and honey with beneficial results in functional impotency, premature ejaculation and thinness of the semen.

Cardamom

This popular spice, known as 'queen of spices', is a sex stimulating food. It is useful in sexual dysfunction like impotency and premature ejaculation. A pinch of powdered cardamom seeds, boiled in milk and sweetened with honey, should be taken every night. It will increase sexual stamina and virility. Excessive use of cardamom should, however, be avoided as it may have adverse effect.

Carrot

This vegetable is an effective aphrodisiac food and is considered beneficial in the treatment of sexual impotence. About 150g of carrots chopped finely, should be taken with a half-boiled egg, dipped in a tablespoon of honey, once daily for a month or two as a sex tonic. This recipe increases sexual stamina.

Cowhage

Cowhage is a famous creeper, which bears flowers and seeds like those of kidney beans. It is a highly aphrodisiac food, which can cure sexual debility and impotency in a short time. One gram of the powder of the fresh root of cowhage should be taken with milk in treating these conditions. It also increases retentivity in copulation.

It is said that if a person holds a piece of the root of this herb of about the thickness of a finger in his mouth during the sexual intercourse, it will check ejaculation of semen as long as he continues to suck the juice.

Regular use of cowhage imparts vigor and vitality. The

seeds of this herb are also beneficial in the treatment of spermatorrhoea or thinness of semen. They are ingredients of several commercial preparations, which are said to have beneficial effects in the management of various sexual disorders.

Dates (dried)

Dried dates are an aphrodisiac food. They are beneficial in the treatment of sexual weakness and impotency. A handful of dates soaked in fresh goat's milk overnight should be ground in the same milk in the morning. A pinch of cardamom powder and honey should be added to this preparation. This makes an effective tonic for improving sex stamina and sterility due to functional disorders. The dried dates, pounded and mixed with almonds and pistachio nuts, forms an effective sex tonic for increasing sexual power.

Drumstick Flowers

The flowers of drumstick tree are an aphrodisiac food. They are valuable in the treatment of sexual debility and impotence. About 15 g of these flowers should be boiled in 250 ml of milk. This makes an effective sex tonic. It is also useful in functional sterility in both males and females.
The powder of the dry bark is also valuable in impotency, premature ejaculation and thinness of semen. About 120 grams of this powder should be boiled in half a litre of water for half an hour. Approximately 30 grams of this mixture, mixed with a tablespoon of honey, should be taken three times daily for a month in treating these conditions.

Fenugreek Seeds

Since ancient times, fenugreek has been held in high

esteem as a tonic for the reproductive system. Pliny, the ancient Roman sage, who wrote a lengthy discourse on spice remedies and quoted many herbal and medical authorities, says that fenugreek, has a beneficial effect on the sex organ. To this day, the Turkish maidens of Tunisia still prepare and eat a mixture of honey and powdered fenugreek seed to improve their feminine figures and sexy appearance.

Fenugreek seeds contain protein and, according to a report in Biological Abstracts, "new free amino acids," the building blocks of the human body. Another substance found in the seeds is trigonelline, which the authoritative U.S. Pharmacopoeia describes as the methylbetaine of nicotinic acid. The seeds also contain aromatic oil similar in composition to cod-liver oil, which is very rich in vitamin D.

The oil contained in fenugreek seed could account for the plant's ancient reputation as a sex rejuvenator for the person deficient in vitamin A and D. For the last several years, the damaging effects on the male organs resulting from vitamin A deficiency in the diet has been under scientific study.

Another possible sex-rejuvenating property contained in fenugreek is trimethylamine. Scientific studies show that it acts as a sex hormone in frogs, causing them to prepare for mating.

Fenugreek can be made into a tea by steeping one teaspoonful of the seeds in a cup of boiling water. However, since heat destroys the enzymes, the full benefits of the seeds' inherent properties are not obtained when the diluted tea form is used. For best results, herbalists suggest adding the seeds in powdered form to foods or fruits and vegetable juices. Alternatively the seeds can be taken in the form of sprouts.

The use of fenugreek seeds is also been found beneficial in the treatment of spermatorrhoea and functional impotency. The seeds should be roasted and two teaspoons should be taken, mixed with equal quantity of powder of the roasted coriander seeds, with milk every night for a month in treating these conditions.

Garlic

Garlic is a natural and harmless powerful aphrodisiac food. Its regular use imparts sexual vigour and vitality. Dr. Robinson, an eminent sexologist of America considers that garlic has a pronounced aphrodisiac effect. It is a tonic for loss of sexual power from any cause and for sexual debility and impotency from over indulgence in sex and nervous exhaustion from dissipating habit. Its use has been found especially valuable for elder persons of high nervous tension and failing sexual power.

Ginger

Ginger is a very valuable sex stimulating food. The juice extracted from this vegetable is considered beneficial in the treatment of sexual weakness. For better results, half a teaspoon of ginger juice should be taken with a half boiled-egg and honey once daily at night for a month. This will tone up the sex centers and cure impotency, premature ejaculation and Spermatorrhoea.

Ginseng

Li-Shih-Chen highly respected oriental physician and pharmacologist, who lived towards the end of the 16th century, hailed ginseng root as an aphrodisiac and prescribed it for a variety of ailments. It is also highly valued in the Far

East as a sex rejuvenator.

The history of this herb shows that it was being used to pep up fading virility by the Chinese men for thousands of years. According to reports coming from the Far East, men who have passed the spring and summer of their lives and use ginseng regularly are able to satisfy their romantic desires as though they were young again. The late Dr. S.N. Chernych of San Francisco was convinced that the Chinese claim for the sex-invigorating power of this ancient wonder-root was true. He said, "Oriental healers are successfully curing patients of sexual impotence, one of the most difficult disorders. I can state from personal experience that the Oriental physicians have cured several men whom I and several other doctors tried to help."

The Chinese healers insist that ginseng does not stimulate the sex glands into unnatural activity but that it is a restorer of the normally healthy sexual function that has become "weary". The potency of ginseng as a sex improver has been confirmed by the Russian scientists, who have been studying the Oriental plant for many years. They have established that the root has a beneficial influence on the sex glands and other endocrine glands. Their findings show that the effects do not lead to premature exhaustion of the organism, for the herb is definitely not a strong stimulant. Russian reports agree with Chinese claims that ginseng act by healthfully invigorating the physiological process.

Ginseng's "sex magic" is not instantaneous. Those who have used the root faithfully over a period of time unanimously agree that its strengthening effect on the reproductive system is slow and gradual. Ginseng can be used in various forms as explained in Chapter 16 on Life-Prolonging Foods.

Honey

The use of honey both as food and as medicine dates from antiquity. It is mentioned frequently in the Bible and in the ancient sacred texts of China, India, Egypt, and Persia. In ancient times, a simple honey potion was said to offer a feeling of rejuvenation. It was prepared by boiling three parts of water to one part honey over a slow fire until two third remained. This honey potion is believed to promote a feeling of rejuvenation and youthful virility. In olden days, the newly married women also drank honey-beer for 30 days to ensure fertility and to guard against female frigidity. It is from this custom the term "honeymoon" is derived. Honey is a spermatogenetic and sex stimulant. Many Asiatics regard it as an aphrodisiac. They believe that it possesses a magical substance, which influences the fertility of women and the virility of men. Honey contains aspartic acid, vitamin E and traces of estrogen, part of the group of female hormones, which are produced by the ovaries that are responsible for female sexuality and development. Honey can be taken mixed in water or milk.

Indian Gooseberry

Indian gooseberry is regarded as a natural rejuvenator. It is said that the great ancient sage Muni Chyawan rejuvenated himself in his late 70's and regained his virility by the use of amla.

This fruit has been credited with aphrodisiac property. This property is attributed to high vitamin C contained in it. Vitamin C boosts energy levels, according to a survey conducted in New York in 1994. Experts say that vitamin C soaks up all those free radicals, which damage healthy cells and make people, feel and look older and less interested in sex. But a diet rich in vitamin C can ward off effects of exposure to infection, tobacco, environmental pollutants, sugar and alcohol. The result is optimal health leading to a better sex life.

Jambul Fruit

This fruit is a specific remedy for spermatorrhoea and sexual debilities. About 200 grams of jambul fruit should be used four times daily for at least a fortnight. This may be followed by one grain of *Sendha Salt*. The quantity of fruit can be increased gradually. This will strengthen sexual organs and the person will gain vigour and vitality.

Lady's Finger

The lady's finger is a very popular table vegetable grown all over India. It is a great sexual tonic. Its regular use increases the sperm cells and thickens the semen. It is mentioned in the ancient Indian literature that the persons who take 5 to 10 grams of root powder of this vegetable with milk and 'mishri' daily, never loose sexual vigour. Those who have deficiency of sperm cells in their semen and also pass undue semen should make liberal use of this vegetable.

Mango

This most popular fruit is a perfect rejuvenative food. Its regular use during the season imparts vigour and vitality and gives exceptional tone to the reproductory system. For better results, the juice of a fully ripe and sweet fibrous mango should be extracted and taken mixed with pure honey.

Musk Melon

This fruit is a sex-strengthening food and its systemic

use has been found especially valuable in rectifying the defects of the seminal fluid. In this mode of treatment, the patient should take an exclusive diet of musk melon for twenty-one days. To begin with, he should take 120 grams of melon at a time for three or four times a day. The quantity of melon may be increased by 10 grams at a time for three days. The maximum quantity should be maintained for two days more and then it should be decreased in the same order.

The pulp of melons only should be consumed. This may be followed by sucking of a piece of sugar candy. The return to normal diet should be gradual, while free use of melons should also be continued. The exclusive diet of musk melon should be concluded by taking fresh fruit and their juices, before resuming the normal diet.

Nutmeg

This popular condiment is an aphrodisiac food. It stimulates sexual desire and serves as medicine in sexual debility and weakness. The powder of nutmeg, mixed with honey and a half-boiled egg, makes an excellent sex tonic. It prolongs the duration of sexual act if taken an hour before conjugal union.

Onion

Onions have been attributed aphrodisiac properties since prehistoric times. They have been hailed as more than food in the Egyptian, Greek, Roman, Arab and Chinese literature. A 16th century Arabic erotic Manuel called 'The Perfumed Garden' written by Sheikh Al Nefzawi, recommends use of the juice of pounded onions mixed with honey to improve sexual power. Onions were considered so potent

234

that in the olden times celibate Egyptian priests were prohibited from eating them. This vegetable is believed to increase libido and strengthen the reproductive organ. In France, newly-weds were fed onion soup in the morning after their wedding night to restore their libido.

A syrup made from onion and honey has been found very effective in restoring sexual. power. This syrup is prepared by mixing 30 grams of onion juice with 60 grams of honey and placing it on fire. It should be taken off the fire when it obtains the consistency of syrup. The patient may take even double the dose if it suits him. It reddens the face within a few days and is one of the best aphrodisiac foods.

Pepper (Black)

This most important spice possesses aphrodisiac property and can be beneficially used in the treatment of sexual impotence. Six peppers with four almonds may be taken once daily with milk in treating this condition. It acts as a nerve-tonic and stimulates sexual desire.

Pumpkin Seeds

Pumpkin seeds are known for their "he-man" power. They have been used for their beneficial effect on the prostate since ancient times. This favorite folk remedy of gypsies, Germans, and others has now drawn the attention of modern scientists.

Dr. W. Devrient of Berlin, Germany, reports that he has been curing patients of prostate trouble by making them eat pumpkin seeds regularly. According to him, this is a disease-preventive food, which contains rejuvenating power for men. Men in Europe and America usually make use of these seeds liberally and remain amazingly free of prostate

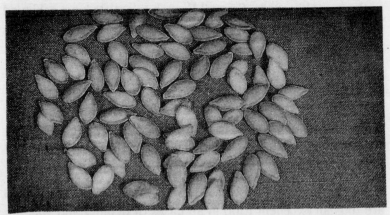

Pumpkin seeds are known for their "he-man" power.

disorders and all its consequences. The prostate gland manufactures prostatic fluid, which nourishes the male spermatozoa and keeps them alive. A new medication, not a drug but a nutrient, which occurs naturally in certain foods, has been successfully used for non-surgical treatment of the enlarged prostate gland. The treatment consists of a mixture of three amino acids-alanine, glycine and glumatic acid. Doctors Julian Grant and Henry Feinblatt, who discovered this important medication, reported that patients with an enlarged prostate associated with urinary difficulties experienced prompt and dramatic relief after taking the amino mixture. Pumpkin seeds contain the very same amino acids that are used in the professional medication.

Chemical analyses of the healthy prostate gland and of spermatozoa show very high concentrations of zinc, whereas the amount of zinc found in the sick prostate is low. It thus seems likely that this mineral is extremely important to the health of the reproductive system. Pumpkin seeds are probably the richest known natural source of zinc. Magnesium is another important mineral found abundantly in the pumpkin seeds. Several French scientists have achieved remarkable results in the prevention and cure of prostatic disorders by administering magnesium compounds.

Raisins (Black)

Raisins are dried grapes. They are esteemed for their high food value, which arises chiefly from their sugar content. They contain eight times more sugar than grapes. A major portion of this sugar is formed by glucose and fruit sugar, which produce quick heat and energy in the body. Raisins are thus an excellent food in all cases of debility and wasting diseases.

Black raisins are regarded as an aphrodisiac food of immense value. They are used for restoration of sexual vigour in Ayurveda. The method for using them for this purpose is to boil them with milk, after washing them thoroughly in tepid water. This will make them swollen and sweet. Eating of such raisins should be followed by the use of milk. Starting with 30 grams of raisins with 200 ml of milk, three times daily, the quantity of raisins should be gradually increased to 50 grams each time.

Safflower Seeds

Safflower seeds are a sex stimulating food. They are highly beneficial in the treatment of sexual debility. For better results, powder of the dry seeds should be mixed with pistachio nuts and almonds. This mixture should be used with milk once before going to bed. It is a very effective aphrodisiac medicine. It improves sexual vigour and thickens semen. It is believed that wearing garments dyed in the juice of the flower of safflower increases sexual desire. In olden days, the newly-weds used to wear such clothes.

Sesame Seeds

Sesame seeds are one of the most important spices grown in the magnificent Hanging Gardens of Babylon. Throughout Babylonian history the seeds were highly valued and their production drew royal attention. The Babylonians loved the nut-like flavor of sesame seeds and used them in various preparations. Women mixed the crushed seeds with honey and ate the delicacy to tone up their sex glands. Dr. Formica of Old Bridge, New Jersey, is reported to have successfully treated scores of married women for what he calls "housewife syndrome," a condition characterised by fatigue, boredom with housework and bedroom "hanky-panky." Sometimes it is accompanied by nervousness, insomnia, headache and backache.

The treatment prescribed by Dr. Formica is a drug, said to be the potassium and magnesium salts of aspartic acid. Dr. Formica reports that he obtained a positive result in 87 per cent of his patients after four to six weeks of treatment with the prescription drug. He claims that the change was astonishing. The women became cheerful, happy, alert and sexually responsive.

A rich supply of potassium and magnesium salts of aspartic acid can be ensured by making a candy of sesame seed and honey. This delicious confection also contains ample amounts of vitamin E, known as fertility vitamin, along with other valuable nutrients like calcium, phosphorus, and unsaturated fatty acids as well as associated lecithin necessary for good health. Sesame seeds also contain 50 per cent more protein than meat.

Dr. Leathem of Rutgers University explains that the hormone hypophyseal produced by the pituitary gland is basically protein in nature and obviously needs this nutrient in the diet for its development. This hormone is a key factor to healthy activity of sex glands.

Wheat Germ Oil

Wheat germ oil is rich in vitamin E and other valuable substances. Research shows that this fine natural product can help boost a woman's femininity and a man's virility. The oil has been reported to induce ovulation in previously barren women and to increase the sperm count in previously sterile men.

Farmers have known, long before science got around to proving it, that vitamin E as contained in wheat germ oil is the fertility factor. They did not call it vitamin E, they just used fresh stone-ground wheat (which contains the wheat germ) and fed it to their magnificent stallions and other animals for breeding purposes. Poultry men also kept insisting that fresh wheat fed to chickens resulted in greater egg production.

Dr. Shute of Canada, renowned for his work on vitamin E and heart disease, has also used the vitamin extensively for reproductive disorders. He reports that experiments conducted on laboratory animals, which were given a diet totally lacking in natural foods containing vitamin E, resulted in derangements of sex life. It produced gradual atrophy of certain generative organs, resulting in the inability to manu-facture sperm and eventually in total sterility. However, before the male organs became completely atrophied, admini-stration of natural vitamin E could restore some sperm activity.

Dr. Shute's success in treating male sterility showed that vitamin E therapy used daily for two weeks increased the sperm count in 48 per cent of the patients, helped 67 per cent to produce only live sperms when they previously had a high proportion or all of their sperms dead, and produced all normal forms in 56 per cent of the men who had abnormal sperms before treatment.

Dr. Shute also reported on the effective results in treating barren women with vitamin E. In a good number of cases, conception took place within a few weeks to several months after vitamin E therapy. Dr Shute reports that wheat germ oil in capsules or bulk, once opened, does not retain its potency much longer than eight weeks even when stored in a refrigerator. Some medical experts believe that wheat germ oil should be taken between meals, when the stomach is reasonably empty. This would ensure that the oil does not get mixed with any rancid fat, which a person may have taken at the mealtime.

CHAPTER 22

ULCER FIGHTING FOODS

Peptic ulcer refers to an eroded lesion in the gastric intestinal mucosa. An ulcer may form in any part of the digestive tract, which is exposed to acid gastric juice, but is usually found in the stomach and the duodenum. The ulcer located in the stomach is known as gastric ulcer and that located in the duodenum is called duodenal ulcer.

Peptic ulcer results from hyperacidity, which is a condition caused by an increase in hydrochloric acid in the stomach. This strong acid, secreted by the cells lining the stomach, affects much of the breakdown of food. It can be potentially dangerous and, under certain circumstances, it may eat its way through the lining of the stomach or duodenum producing, first, irritation of the stomach wall and eventually an ulcer.

Some fascinating discoveries have recently been made by British and Indian researchers as to how food and food constituents strengthen the stomach's resistance to harmful ulcer-producing juices. Thus, British investigators detected a 20 per cent thicker stomach lining in animals' fed with powder made from plantains, the banana-like fruit. Indian researchers photographed the rejuvenation of ulcerated cells in guinea pigs. The healing has resulted from the increased mucins, substances that shield the stomach lining from damage, produced by drinking cabbage juice.

Thus, one way foods can fight ulcers is by strengthening the stomach lining so that it is not easily eaten away by the attacks from acids. Certain foods accomplish this by stimulating the proliferation of cells in the stomach lining. This triggers rapid release of mucus, which cover the cells with a protective coating, thereby sealing them off from harmful effects of acids.

Further, anti-bacterial foods such as curd or yoghurt, cabbage and liquorice may serve as more appropriate medicines for ulcers and gastritis, an inflammation of the stomach lining, than previously thought. This is because the scientists have discovered that a microbe known as *H. Pylori* appears to be a cause of peptic ulcer in many cases. Ulcer treatment now often includes antibiotics. Anti-bacterial foods may thus also help in curing ulcer.

FOODS THAT FIGHT STOMACH ULCERS
Almond Milk, Ash Gourd, Banana and Plantain, Cabbage Juice, Fenugreek Seeds, Fiber-Rich Foods, Garlic, Ladys' Finger or Okra, Lime, Liquorice and Wood Apple.

Almond Milk
Milk prepared from almonds possesses anti-ulcer property. It is considered beneficial in the treatment of both gastric and duodenal ulcers. It binds the excess of acid in the stomach and supplies high quality protein. Almond milk is prepared by grinding the blanched almonds to a smooth paste and adding cold boiled water to the consistency of the milk. With the addition of little honey, it makes a delicious and nutritious drink. One kilogram of milk may be obtained from 250 grams of almonds.

Ash Gourd

Ash gourd, also known as white gourd or wax gourd, is an ash-coloured, large-fruited type vegetable like pumpkin. It is a nutritive and wholesome vegetable. It is an anti-ulcer food. The dilute juice of this vegetable is highly beneficial in the treatment of peptic ulcer. This juice is prepared by adding equal quantity of water to juice of ash gourd squeezed out after grating the raw vegetable. A glass of this juice should be taken daily in the morning on an empty stomach. Foods of all sorts should be avoided for about two or three hours afterwards. This will also relieve inflammation with swelling anywhere in the alimentary canal.

Banana and Plantain

Banana and plantain, the large banana-like fruits, are staple in many tropical countries. They are of great value as an ulcer fighting foods. These fruits possess anti-ulcer property and have long been used in folk medicine to treat ulcers. Indian physicians often prescribe dried powder made from green plantains, to treat ulcers. The success of this treatment is reported to be 70 per cent.

According to British Pharmacist Dr. Ralph Best at the University of Aston in Birmingham, banana stimulate proliferation of cells and mucus that form a stronger barrier between the stomach lining and destructive or eroding acid. In fact, when animals were fed banana powder, researchers observed a visible thickening of the stomach wall. In one Australian test, rats were fed bananas and then high amounts of acid to induce ulcers. They suffered very little stomach damage. The bananas prevented 75 per cent of the expected ulceration.

Banana and milk are considered an ideal diet for the ulcer

patients who are in an advanced state of the disease. Dr. A.M. Conell, an eminent nutritionist, discovered that a ripe banana contains serotonin, a chemical which has a marked effect on the excessive secretion of hydrochloric acid in the stomach, which usually results in gastric ulcer and gastritis. In such condition when banana is given with milk, the acid is neutralized by the action of serotonin. The pectin present in banana acts as a mechanical barrier by coating over the inflamed surface and vitamin C helps heal the ulcer quickly. One more advantage of pectin is that it prevents the absorption of toxins produced by the pathogenic organisms by covering the naked surface in the gastro-intestinal tract. Banana also affords a protection against ulcers produced by stress situation.

When plantains are used for treating ulcers, they must be cooked before eating, because they are too hard and tough to eat in raw form. Green plantains are considered more potent medicine for healing ulcers than ripe ones.

Cabbage Juice

Cabbage contains anti-ulcer compounds. It can help heal ulcers. This has been revealed by the experiments conducted by Dr. Garnet Cheney, M.D., a professor of Medicine at Stanford University School of Medicine, in the 1950s. He demonstrated that just over 850 ml. of fresh cabbage juice every day relieved pain and healed both gastric and duodenal ulcers better and faster than standard medical treatments. In a test, he made 55 patients drink cabbage juice. About 95 per cent felt better within two to five days. X-rays and gastroscopy revealed a rapid healing of gastric ulcers in only one-quarter of the average time. The duodenal ulcers of patients who were given cabbage juice also healed in one-third the usual time.

Cabbage juice appears to act by strengthening the stomach lining's resistance to acid attacks. Cabbage contains gefarnate, a compound used as an anti-ulcer drug, as well as a chemical that resembles carbenoxolone, another sparingly used anti-ulcer drug. Essentially, the drugs incites cells to draw out a thin mucus barrier as a shield against acid attacks.

Dr. G. B. Singh, of Central Drug Research Institute in Lucknow, induced ulcers in guinea pigs and cured them with cabbage juice. During the healing, he took extensive microscopic photos of the cell changes. These changes revealed that cabbage juice generated increased mucus activity that rejuvenated ulcerated cells leading to healing. To render the juice more palatable, Dr. Cheney often mixed celery juice, extracted both from stalk and greens, with pineapple juice, tomato juice or citrus juice. Chilling the mixed juice also helps improve the flavor. The juice, however, should not be taken all at once, but at many intervals throughout the day. If one does not have a juicer or blender, one can nibble on raw cabbage four or five times a day.

Fenugreek Seeds

Fenugreek seeds possess anti-ulcer property. They are highly effective in the treatment of peptic ulcers. A tea made from these seeds soothes inflamed stomach and intestine and cleanses the stomach. It helps healing of ulcers as the mild coating of mucilaginous material deposited by fenugreek seeds, as it passes through the stomach and intestines, provides a protective shell for the ulcers.

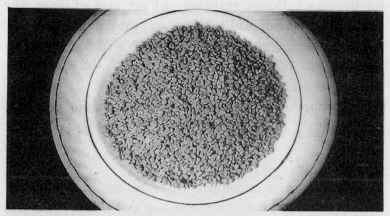

Fenugreek seeds are highly effective in the treatment of peptic ulcers.

Fibre-Rich Foods

It has long been recommended that the low-fibre bland diet relieves or prevents ulcers. Contrary to this view, it is now believed that a lack of roughage, far from discouraging ulcers, encourages them. In support of this belief, Dr. Frank I. Tovey, M.D., a surgeon at the University College of London and a prominent researcher on diet and ulcers, points out that the Japanese, who eat heavy diet of polished rice, have the highest peptic ulcer rate in the world. Ulcers are also a major problem in the rice eating areas of Southern India. But they are rare in North India where *chapattis* or unrefined wheat breads are the staple food. This is also true in China, where ulcers are prevalent in the southern rice growing areas and less so in the northern wheat raising lands, he says.

Further, taking a high-fibre diet seems to help heal ulcers and prevent relapses. In Bombay, Dr. S. L. Malhotra took up a study on a group of 42 patients with healed ulcers who were regular rice eaters. He had half of them convert to a Punjabi type unrefined wheat diet. He followed them for five years. During that time, 81 per cent of those who consumed rice only had relapses and their ulcers flared up again. In comparison, only 14 per cent of the high-fibre wheat eaters had a recurrence of ulcers. Fibre seems to have a protective effect and it reduces gastric acid concentrations. It might irritate the stomach lining and make it tough.

Garlic

This pungent condiment possesses anti ulcer property. It may help retard stomach damage and ulcers. This was discovered by researchers at Catholic University Medical College in Seoul, Korea. They fed rats doses of alcohol aimed at harming the stomach lining. Some animals also got pure garlic or garlic compounds. The rats who got the garlic and components had much less stomach damage, especially less haemorrhaging and cell destruction beneath the surface of the lining. Researchers attributed the protection not to the inhibiting property of gastric acid secretion, but to mild irritation that excited production of protective hormone like substances that strengthened stomach lining resistance.

Lady's Finger or Okra

Lady's finger is considered to be an anti-ulcer food. It is one of the most effective remedies for peptic ulcer. According to Dr. J. Meyer and his associates, powdered okra is an efficient means of speedily relieving the pain of peptic ulcer. Modern investigations show that the pain of peptic ulcer is not directly due to the chemical effects of an over abundant gastric juice, but to spasm or cramp of the pylorus, due to irritation of the sensitive duodenum by the acid gastric contents. The emollient okra protects the sensitive duodenal surfaces and so stops the cramps. The mucilage of lady's finger is especially valuable in treating the burning sensation in the stomach caused by peptic ulcer. It can be extracted from this vegetable by cutting four capsules into 2.5cm pieces and boiling them in 225ml of water for about 15 minutes. After cooling, the pieces are squeezed and the mucilage is extracted and strained through a muslin cloth. A tablespoon of honey and pinch of rock salt is added to this mucilage and is used once daily as a cure for this condition.

Lime

Lime is food of great value in treating peptic ulcer. The citric acid in this fruit has an alkaline reaction in the system. This acid, together with the mineral salts present in the juice, helps the digestion by assisting the absorption of fats and alcohol and by neutralising excessive bile produced by the liver. The juice counteracts the effects of greasy food and reduces gastric acidity.

Liquorice

Liquorice possesses anti ulcer property. According to Dr. James Duke, Ph.D. and Botanist at the U.S. Department of Agriculture, liquorice is highly beneficial in the treatment of peptic ulcer. He says that numerous studies have attributed liquorice root with formidable antiulcer properties. For instance, Scandinavian scientists found that liquorice compounds reduced acids, stimulated mucus secretion and helped stomach wall cells repair themselves.

Pharmaceutical companies have even developed a drug called Caved-S-which is essentially liquorice without its most troublesome ingredient, glycrrhizin. In a British test of 100 ulcer patients, the liquorice drug, which is chewed, was just as effective as the commonly used ulcer drug Tagamet in healing ulcers.

Liquorice is especially useful in the removal of pain due to stomach ulcers. The demulcent action of this condiment decreases the irritation due to acids. Pieces of the dry root soaked overnight in water and the infusion taken with rice gruel greatly helps in treating ulcers.

Continuous and uninterrupted use of liquorice in the treatment of stomach ulcer is however not advisable, as it may cause increase in weight and puffiness of body. It should also be avoided in pregnancy and in deseased heart and kidney conditions.

Wood Apple

Wood apple is a spherical whitish fruit, with hard woody pericarp and aromatic pulp. The tree is spiny and contains feather-like leaves and reddish flowers. The leaves

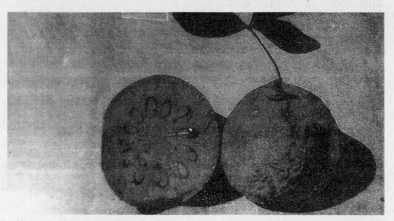

The use of woodapple leaves has been found beneficial in the treatment of both gastric and duodenal ulcers.

of the tree are aromatic and possess astringent and carminative properties.

The leaves also possess anti ulcer property. Their use has
been found beneficial in the treatment of both gastric and
duodenal ulcers. An infusion of the leaves should be taken
to treat this condition. This infusion is prepared by soaking
overnight 15 g of the leaves in 250 ml of water. In the
morning this water should be strained and taken as a drink.
The pain and discomfort will be relieved when this treatment
is continued for a few weeks. The leaves are rich in tannins,
which reduce inflammation and help healing ulcers.

CHAPTER 23

WEIGHT-REDUCING FOODS

Proper weight control is of utmost importance in the maintenance of good health. Obesity may be described as a bodily condition characterised by excessive deposition or storage of fat in adipose tissue. It usually results from consumption of food in excess of physiological needs.

Obesity is a serious health hazard as the extra fat puts a strain on the heart, kidneys and liver as well as the large weight-bearing joints such as the hips, knees and ankles, which ultimately shortens the life span. Over weight persons are susceptible to several diseases like coronary thrombosis, heart failure, high blood pressure, diabetes, arthritis, gout, liver and gall bladder disorders.

Diet plays a dominant role in any weight reduction programme. There are specific foods, which contain certain compounds found helpful in weight reduction.

FOODS THAT REDUCE BODY WEIGHT
Banana, Cabbage, Fennel, Finger Millet, Jujube Leaves, Lecithin, Lemon, Lime, Low-Salt Food and Tomato.

Banana

A ripe banana mashed in plain cow's milk, mixed with a tablespoon of fresh banana flower juice, is an excellent weight-reducing food. This mixture should be taken two to three times a day for treating obesity. Sweets and fried foods should, however, be completely eliminated from the diet. This recipe is quite effective if used for a couple of months. It helps the weight reduction by supplying low calories, increasing urinary output and washing out the extra sodium chloride from the body.

Cabbage

This popular green leafy vegetable is of great value as a weight reducing food. Recent research has discovered in cabbage a valuable content called tartronic acid, which inhibits the conversion of sugar and other carbohydrates into fat. A helping of cabbage salad would be the simplest way to stay slim and a painless way of dieting.

A hundred grams of cabbage yield only 27 kilocalories of energy, while the same quantity of wheat bread will yield about 240 calories. Cabbage is found to posses the maximum biological value with minimum calorific value. Moreover, it gives a lasting feeling of fullness in the stomach and is easily digestible.

Fennel

This popular culinary spice is credited with the property to reduce weight since ancient times. The ancient Greeks were well acquainted with the weight-reducing power of this herb, as the Greek name for fennel is *Marathron*, which is derived from *Mariano*, meaning "to grow thin". An eminent nutritionist William Coles used seeds, leaves and roots of garden fennel in drinks and broths for those who were over weight. It helped greatly in reducing their unmanageable weight and made them grow thin and slender. The best way to take fennel for the purpose of reducing weight is in the form of tea made from fennel seeds. This tea is prepared by putting four teaspoons of the seeds in one litres of boiling water and allowing them to simmer for five minutes. The container should be kept covered and allowed to stand for 15 minutes and then strained. One cupful of this tea should be taken three or four times daily.

Finger Millet

Finger millet is a weight reducing food. It is an ideal food for the obese because its digestion is slow and due to this the carbohydrate takes longer time to get absorbed. By eating *ragi*-preparations, the constant desire to eat gets curbed, thereby reducing the daily caloric intake. At the same time, it supplies abundant calcium, phosphorus, iron, vitamin B1 and B2 and prevents malnutrition in spite of restricted food.

Jujube Leaves

The leaves of jujube or Indian plum are a valuable food in reducing weight. A handful of leaves should be soaked overnight in water and this water should be taken in the morning, preferably on an empty stomach. This treatment should be continued for at least one month to achieve beneficial results.

Lecithin

The use of lecithin, a fatty food substance, mostly extracted from soyabean, is of great importance in any weight reduction programme. It helps control weight by pulling fat deposits from fat bulges in the body and burning them out. It also helps a person feel well fed on less food intake so that he is not tempted to overeat or nibble between meals. Lecithin is available in the form of capsules, granules or liquids. Foods rich in lecithin, besides soyabean, are vegetable oils, whole grain cereals and unpasteurised milk.

Lemon

This citrus fruit is a valuable food for reducing weight. Substantial reduction in weight can be achieved by taking an exclusive diet of lemon juice. In this mode of treatment, the obese person should be given nothing except plenty of water on the first day. On the second day, he should take juice of three lemons, mixed with equal amount of water. One lemon should be subsequently increased each day until the juice of 12 lemons is consumed per day. Then the number of lemons should be reduced in the same order until three lemons are taken in a day. The patient may feel weak and hungry on first two days, but afterwards the condition will stabilise by itself.

Lime

The juice of lime is an excellent food medicine for weight reduction. Fasting on lime juice honey water has been found beneficial in the treatment of obesity without the loss of energy and appetite. In this mode of treatment, one spoon of fresh honey should be mixed with a juice of half a lime in a glass of lukewarm water and taken at regular intervals.

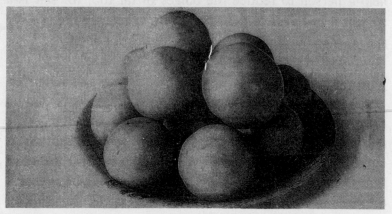

The juice of lime is an excellent food medicine for weight reduction.

Low-Salt Food

Restricting salt is an easy way to slim. Salt attracts and holds water in the body. Thus for instance, just one teaspoonful of salt, will retail three litres of water in the tissues of the body. So if a person wishes to lose weight with very little efforts, he should take as little salt as possible. This may help him shed as much as one and half kg in the first week. He should also avoid foods that have been salted such as potato chips, salted peanuts, salted crackers, salted cheeses and foods that are preserved in salt like pickles, relishes and certain types of sausages.

The obese person should also avoid water softened artificially because of its high sodium content. The body can get all the vital food salts it needs for well being from fruits and vegetables in their natural state.

Salt also makes a person thirsty and hence he drinks more water, which means more weight. A person can carry four and half to seven litres of water due to the salt that is in the body. When a person gives up the salt habit he will shed liquid weight, not fat. However, eliminating salt will greatly help a person to reduce the bulges of fat too, for salt is a stimulant and excites the appetite by increasing the flow of saliva, thereby creating a greater desire for food.

Tomato

This vegetable fruit is also very valuable food in reducing weight. One or two ripe tomatoes taken early morning, without breakfast, for a couple of months is considered a safe method of weight reduction, at the same time supplying the essential food elements which preserve the health.

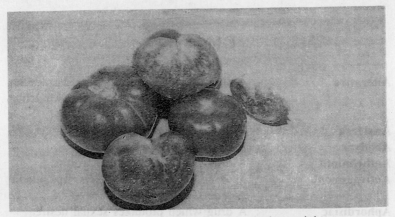

Tomatoes are a valuable food in reducing weight.

Glossary

Alterative : A drug which corrects disordered processes of nutrition and restores the normal function of an organ or of the system.

Analgesic : A drug which alleviates pain.

Anodyne : A drug that relieves pain.

Anthelmintic : A drug that kills intestinal worms.

Antispasmodic : A drug which counteracts spasmodic disorders.

Aphordisiac : A drug which promotes sexual desire.

Astringent : A drug which arrests secretion or bleeding.

Camphor : A White, translucent, crystalline, swiftly evaporating substance with an aromatic smell.

Carminative : A drug which relieves flatulence by expelling wind from the stomach.

Decanted : Gradually poured from one container to another, without disturbing the sediment.

Decoction : A process of boiling down so as to extract some essence.

Demulcent : An agent that exercises a soothing effect on the skin and mucous membranes.

Diaphoretic : A drug that induces copious perspiration.

Diuretic : A drug which increases the secretion and discharge of urine.

DNA : A genetic material of cells.

Emulsion : A fine dispersion of fatty liquid in another liquid, usually water.

Endocrine glands : Glands secreting directly into the blood stream—also known as ductless glands.

Expectorant : A drug that promotes the removal of catarrhal matter and phlegm from the bronchial tubes.

Haemorrhage : Bleeding, especially profuse, from any part of the body.

Heartburn : A burning feeling in the regions of the chest and stomach, generally due to indigestion.

Hepatitis	: Inflammation of the liver.
Infusion	: A liquid obtained by steeping the herb, and the likes in liquid to extract the content.
Insulin	: A hormone produced in the pancreas by the islets of langherhans, regulating the amount of glucose in the blood and the lack of which causes diabetes.
Jaundice	: A disease characterised by yellow discoloration of the skin and the tissues due to deposition in them of the pigment bilirubin.
Laxative	: A drug which produces evacuated bowels.
Lumbago	: A disease marked by severe pain in Lower part of the back.
Malaria	: An infection with parasite of malaria, marked by recurrent shivering, rise in temperature and general aching of the body.
Malic acid	: An organic acid found in unripe apples and other fruits.
Measles	: An infectious febrile disease, marked by a cold in the head, running of the eyes and nose and appearance of white tiny spots on the inner side of the cheek and of rash all over the body.
Micturition	: Urination.
Migraine	: Periodic attack of headache affecting one side of the head.
Mucilage	: A sticky substance extracted from certain plants.
Mumps	: An infectious disease marked by the inflammation of the salivary glands.
Narcotic	: A drug which induces deep sleep.
Neuralgia	: Pain felt along a nerve.
Otitis	: Inflammation of the ear.
Paralysis	: A disease in which there is loss of power of voluntary movement in any part of the body.
Pharyngitis	: Inflammation of the pharynx.
Piles	: An inflamed condition of the veins in the rectal region.

Poultice	:	A soft, medicated and usually heated mass applied to the body and kept in place with muslin, for relieving soreness and inflammation.
Pneumonia	:	Inflammation of the lungs.
Pulmonary	:	Pertaining to the lungs.
Rhizomes	:	An underground root like stem bearing both roots and shoots.
Rubefacient	:	A mild counter irritant.
Scitica	:	An inflammation of the scitic nerve at the back of the thigh.
Sedative	:	A drug which reduces excitement, irritation and pain.
Tannic acid	:	A complex natural organic compound of a yellowish colour used as an astrigent.
Tannin	:	An astingent chemical substance found in tea, coffee and the barks of some trees.
Ulcer	:	An open sore on the skin.
Uric acid	:	A crystalline acid forming constituent of urine.
Wart	:	A hypertrophy of or growth on the skin.
Whooping cough	:	An acute infectious disease characterised by peculiar spasmodic attacks of coughing.

ENGLISH	HINDI	BENGALI	GUJRATI	KAN
Tamarind	Imli	Tetul	Amli	Hunis
Tomato	Tamator	Tamater	Tameton	Toma
Turmeric	Haldi	Holud	Haldi	Anas
Valerian	Jalakan	—	—	—
Walnuts	Akhrot	Akhrot	Akhrot	—
Watercress	chandrasur	Chandrasana	Asalia	Alvi
Watermelon	Tarbuz	Tarmuj	Tarbuj	Kalla
Wood apple	Kaith	Kath bel	Kothu	Bele

NADA	MALAYALAM	MARATHI	TAMIL	TELUGU
e Ambli	Puli	Chinch	Puli	Chintha Amlika
o	Thakkali	Velvangi	Semi—tekkali	Seemavankay
ina	Manjal	Halad	Manjal	Pasupu
	—	Kalavala	—	—
	—	Akhrod	—	—
	Thutta—kaya—kami—kal	Ahliv	Alli ilai	Aditayalu
gadi	Thannir mathan	Kalingad	Darbusini	puchakayi
	Narivilia Vilampazham	—	Narivilia Vilampazham	Velaga

Bibliography

1. Jean Carper, *Food Your Miracle Medicine*, London, Simon & Schuster, first edition, 1995.
2. Bakhru H.K., *Natural Home Remedies for Common Ailments*, New Delhi, Orient Paperbacks, sixth printing 1999.
3. Bakhru H.K., *Herbs That Heal*, New Delhi, Orient Paperbacks, Tenth Printing 1998.
4. Bakhru H.K., *Foods that Heal*, New Delhi, Orient Paperbacks, Fifteenth Printing 1999.
5. Paul Bergner, *Healing Power of Garlic*, New Delhi, Orient Paperback 1998.
6. Oscar. Prof. Dr. Aman, *Medicinal Secrets of Your Food*, Mysore, Indo-American Hospital, First Edition 1985.
7. Kvj. Ganapati Singh Verma, *Miracles of Fruits*, New Delhi, The Rasayan Pharmacy, 9th Edition 1978.
8. Kvj. Ganpati Singh Verma, *Miracles of Indian Herbs*, New Delhi, Rasayan Pharmacy, Third Reprint 1982.
9. Kvj. Ganapati Singh Verma, *Miracles of Honey*, New Delhi, The Rasayan Pharmacy, First Edition 1984.
10. Kvj. Ganapati Singh Verma, *Miracles of Onion*, New Delhi, The Rasayan Pharmacy, First Edition 1981.
11. P.E. Norris, *About Honey*, Northamptonshire, Thorsons Publishers Limited, Sixth Edition 1981.
12. P.E. Norris, *About Yogurt*, Northamptonshire, Thorsons Publishers Limited, Third Edition 1980.
13. Ceres Esplan, *Herbal Teas*, Northamptonshire, Thorsons Publishers Limited, Third Edition 1986.
14. Carlson Wade, *Health Secrets of Orient*, New Delhi, Allied Publishers Private Limited.
15. Lucas Richard, *The Magic of Herbs in Daily Living*, New York, Parker Publishing House 1972.
16. S.J. Singh, *Food Remedies*, Lucknow, Nature Cure Council of Medical
17. William L. Esser, *Dictionary of Natural Foods*, Bridgeport, Natural Hygiene Press, 1983.

INDEX

DR. BHAKHRU'S OTHER BESTSELLERS WITH JAICO

A Complete Handbook of Nature Cure (Revised & Enlarged Edition)

This revised and enlarged Handbook is a most comprehensive family guide to health the natural way. Author makes a compelling ease, for treating diseases through natural methods which rely on natural foods, natural elements, yoga and observance of other laws of nature. This well illustrated book is no doubt beneficial for those who desire good health through the use of natural remedies. The book also contains numerous food charts to enable the readers to plan their daily diet for good health.

In view of its valuable contents, this book has been awarded first prize under the category Primer on Naturopathy For Healthy Living by the Jury of Judges. This prize was given at "Book Prize Award Scheme" for the year 1997-1998 instituted by the National Institute of Naturopathy, an autonomous body under Government of India, Ministry of Health and Family Welfare.

Diet Cure for Common Ailments

Book covers the whole gamut of ailments which can be cured merely by proper food habits and regulation of one's life, without recourse to medicinal treatment. The book is based on the theories and fundamentals of Nature Cure that go to preserve health and vitality and regain these when lost. It is a useful guid to those who wish to treat themselves through this system at home.

A Handbook of Natural Beauty

This book is every woman's guide to Looking Good, Feeling Good and Staying Fit. It enlightens readers on:
- Which foods make you fairer
- Why water will do more for you than any skin cream

- A delicious way to prevent tooth decay
- How to prevent your hair from falling and greying and a natural hair dye
- Exercises for a healthier, lovelier you and ..... a lot more.

Nature Cure for Children's Diseases

This book gives all essential tips you require to put your "little one". at ease. It is an alternative way out to treat your child and keep the doctor at bay. It helps you discover:

- What to do when worms infest your child's tummy
- What to do when lice swarm all over your child's head
- How to give a hot water enema
- How to apply mud packs
- How to give a massage and ..... a lot more.

Naturopathy For The Elderly

The book deals with diseases commonly prevalent in the elderly and prescribes time-tested nature cure methods for their treatment. It contains invaluable nature cure methods which if practised sincerely can work miracles for probems related with ageing viz. poor health, loss of functions, slower mental faculties and development of other frightening diseases.

Indian Spices And Condiments As Natural Healers

Spices and condiments are one of the most important forms of natural foods. Besides culinary uses, they have been used in indigenous system of medicine as natural healers since ancient times. They thus form part of our heritage healing. This book describes in great detail the medicinal virtues of different specific spices and condiments, and their usefulness in the treatment of various common ailments. This information can serve as a guide to the readers to solve their common health problems through the use of specific spices and condiments, besides adopting a well-balanced natural diet.

❀ ❀ ❀